SLIP AND FALL PREVENTION

A Practical Handbook

SLIP AND FALL PREVENTION

A Practical Handbook

Steven Di Pilla, ARM, AIC
ESIS, Inc.

LEWIS PUBLISHERS

A CRC Press Company
Boca Raton London New York Washington, D.C.

Library of Congress Cataloging-in-Publication Data

Di Pilla, Steven.
Slip and fall prevention : a practical handbook / by Steven Di Pilla
p. cm.
Includes bibliographical references and index.
ISBN 1-56670-659-9 (alk. paper)
1. Industrial safety. 2. Falls (Accidents)--Prevention. I. Title.

T55.D565 2003
620.8′6—dc21 2003046640

Direct all inquiries to CRC Press LLC, 2000 N.W. Corporate Blvd., Boca Raton, Florida 33431.

Lewis Publishers is an imprint of CRC Press LLC

No claim to original U.S. Government works
International Standard Book Number 1-56670-659-9
Library of Congress Card Number 2003046640
Printed in the United States of America 1 2 3 4 5 6 7 8 9 0
Printed on acid-free paper

Foreword

Walking is nothing more than the successive loss and recovery of balance -

A. Sussman
R. Goode

THE MAGIC OF WALKING

How seemingly simple, on the surface, the subject of pedestrian safety with respect to slips, trips, and falls appears. Everyone at one time or another has probably experienced both a trip and a slip and the subsequent fall. The embarrassment of the experience, and what we perceive as looking like a fool, tends to make us get up as quickly as possible and flee the scene, hoping that no one saw the buffoonery we just committed. Fortunately, some individuals among us are young and agile enough to suffer little from such circumstances. No report of the fall is ever made, and the occurrence is somewhat akin to the proverbial tree in the forest that crashes to the ground (i.e., If no one saw the fall, then was there really a fall?). Falls are notoriously underreported. Yet the falls that do occur, and that are reported, have a significant impact on our society and its safety, health, and welfare. The statistics attributed to fall injuries leave no question that falls are a significant problem and concern.

As research in the field of pedestrian safety marches on, we gain more knowledge in kinesiology, tribology, and biomechanics. However, the gains lead us to the realization that the things that we do know are outweighed by the things that we do not know. The measurement of slip resistance has evolved from the beanbag-and-scale experiment, to the Hunter Machine, to the James Machine, and beyond. Certain schools of thought do not like change and hold onto the past with complete disregard for technological advancement, while others continue the pursuit for a better way — a way that models, as closely as is possible, the interacting forces between the foot and ground in the presence of contaminants, and quantitatively relates to what the human foot encounters during ambulation. This quest is not about to end soon. Nothing can ever be measured or studied perfectly, and there will always be room for improvement, even after we think we have gotten close to perfection.

In the midst of many ongoing debates, Steven Di Pilla has gathered the most current and relevant information available, and compiled this guide as an information resource in order to provide the reader with simple, proven, and effective knowledge as well as the means to reduce fall occurrences. Understanding why falls occur serves as a foundation for mitigating falls. Many books are available on this subject, with most focusing on "slips and falls." This volume covers the gamut, from slips to stumbles to trips. From a safety engineering perspective, it is invaluable because it covers the four engineering priorities of dealing with hazards: elimination of the hazard through design; guarding the hazard; warning of the hazard; and training to minimize the risk of the hazard.

As a colleague of Mr. Di Pilla, I can attest to his competence and to what I believe is his overall objective: the reduction of injuries due to slips, trips, stumbles, and falls. Mr. Di Pilla is the first professional I have ever encountered in the risk and insurance industry who looks at risk from a proactive perspective, instead of the typical reactive one. Risk management is a tool that many in the industry unfortunately use to fend off exposure and responsibility by passing the risk off to others through indemnity and assumed risk. Steve Di Pilla is of a different breed of professional, with certain gifts that most of us do not possess. I could go on and on about his qualities and his expertise in this area. Suffice it to say that, to my knowledge, he has put together the most comprehensive reference resource on the subject of pedestrian safety.

Slip and Fall Prevention: A Practical Guide is a tool to be used and referenced by safety professionals, engineers, architects, maintenance organizations, property managers and owners, and anyone else who is interested in reducing the occurrence of falls. The citations, references, links, and forms are intended to assist in the development of a fall-prevention program, or to improve an already existing one. Mr. Di Pilla has done us all a great service in providing this up-to-date and comprehensive reference guide.

Keith Vidal, P.E.
Vidal Engineering, LLC

Preface

This publication is intended as a reference for use by safety practitioners in assessing the exposure of slips and falls, reducing the potential for falls, and minimizing the severity of fall accidents. The following areas are covered:

Introduction: This provides a framework for the scope of the problem, various statistics regarding fall occurrences, and populations at risk.

Chapter 1 — Physical Evaluation: This chapter deals with standards and guidelines relating to the design and layout aspects of a facility, including such areas as traffic flow, level walking surfaces, parking areas, changes in levels, stairways, handrails, ramps, entrances and exits, and the impact of ice/snow.

Chapter 2 — Management Controls: As important as facility design is the related operational controls developed and implemented to maintain and complement good layout and design. This chapter addresses the less tangible features of slip and fall prevention and mitigation, such as spill and wet programs, self-inspection, construction/special event control, lighting, and contractual arrangements.

Chapter 3 — Principles of Slip Resistance: To effectively assess, improve, and maintain good slip resistance, it is first necessary to understand the fundamentals and special considerations in traction measurement and control. Included in this chapter is information on slip resistance factors, a history of the often-cited 0.5 threshold, an overview of key factors such as surface roughness and wet testing, and classes of tribometers.

Chapter 4 — ASTM Standards Related to Pedestrian Safety: ASTM International, formerly the American Society for Testing and Materials, now is the premier developer of pedestrian safety-related standards in the U.S. To conduct valid and reliable testing, it is essential to be familiar with the advantages and disadvantages of tribometer test methods. Discussed in this part of the text are the current state of ASTM tribometer and pedestrian safety standards, profiles of each ASTM test method and apparatus, test pad materials, and plans for the set of ASTM "gold" standards in slip resistance.

Chapter 5 — Other U.S. Standards and Guidelines: Other federal and consensus standards-making organizations have developed standards relating to slip resistance. Understanding the background, intent, and practical use of these documents can be an important reference tool. This chapter reviews the slip resistance specifications from UL, OSHA, ADA, Access Board, NFPA, Federal and Military Specifications, and ANSI.

Chapter 6 — Flooring and Tribometry: Practical applications of tribometry are covered in this chapter, including equipment maintenance and calibration essentials, establishing competency qualifications for tribometer operators, identification of flooring materials, and the impact of factors such as wear and cleaning methodologies.

Chapter 7 — Footwear: The design, selection, and maintenance of footwear are essential considerations for an effective footwear program in the workplace. Footwear programs provide an additional area of slip and fall control for employers.

Chapter 8 — Overseas Slip Resistance Standards: As businesses expand to encompass operations all over the world, it becomes more relevant to gain an understanding of slip resistance protocols and standards outside of the U.S. This chapter discusses the differences in approaches to this subject, along with the more prevalent test methods including ramp tests, pendulum testers, and digitized dragsled devices, as well as a discussion of overseas organizations involved in slip resistance research.

Chapter 9 — Profiles of Selected Industries: Whereas many types of businesses have lesser exposures to pedestrian falls, others have higher than average loss experience. This chapter provides a snapshot of the special hazards and recommended controls of high-risk operations such as restaurants, hotels/motels, health care, and retail/mercantile facilities.

Chapter 10 — Accident Investigation and Mitigation: Prevention measures cannot eliminate all losses. To handle fall accidents effectively, proper investigation and mitigation controls must be in place. This includes gathering the needed information, investigating the facts, providing prompt and courteous aid to the injured, and combating fraudulent cases.

Acknowledgments

The author thanks the following individuals for their valuable contributions: John S. Ingram, vice-president of risk control services at ESIS, Inc., for the faith, support, and commitment to complete this book. William English, president of William English Inc., for getting me started and for his encouragement in this line of research. Dan Schultz, ASTM International staff manager to Committee F-13, for helping to guide me through the maze of standard development both domestically and overseas. David Fleisher, vice-president of Consulting Engineers and Scientists, for continuing to demonstrate unshakable (if implausible) confidence in my abilities. Henry Shable, senior risk control specialist for ESIS, Inc., for authoring the chapter on industry-specific fall prevention (Chapter 9, "Profiles of Selected Industries").

The Author

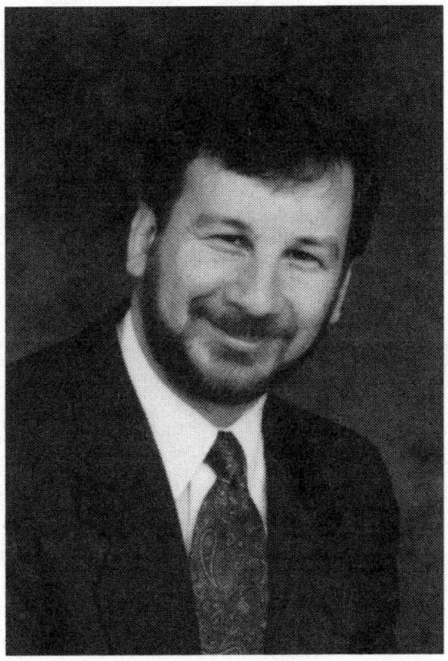

Steven Di Pilla is the director of product research and development for risk control services at ESIS, Inc., an ACE USA[1] risk management service company. He is responsible for identifying and filling the needs of staff consultants, researching technical issues and developing references, training and certification programs, standards, loss analyses, and external publications. He began his career at the former CIGNA Property & Casualty, now part of ACE USA, in 1980.

A professional member of the American Society of Safety Engineers (ASSE) and the ASSE Standards Development Committee, he currently serves as chairman of American Society of Testing and Materials (ASTM) Technical Committee F13 Safety and Traction for Footwear and is former chairman of subcommittee F13.10 — Traction. Other ASTM committee membership includes C21 Ceramics, D01 Paints, D21 Polishes, F06 Resilient Flooring, F08 Sports Equipment and Facilities, F15 Consumer Products, and E34 Safety and Health. He also serves as chairman of the American National Standards Institute (ANSI) 1264.2, which deals with the slip resistance of working/walking surfaces, and is a member of Underwriters Laboratories STP 410, dealing with the measurement of slip resistance of walkway surfaces.

Di Pilla is an active member of numerous other professional organizations including: the Inland Marine Underwriters Association, Loss Prevention Committee (former chairman); the American Society for Industrial Security (ASIS); the World Safety Organization (vice president, New Jersey Chapter); and the National Fire Protection Association (NFPA) Means of Egress Committee for Safety to Life, and the Cultural Resources Committee. He is the author of numerous studies and articles, and has presented extensively.

Di Pilla holds a B.B.A. in Property & Casualty Insurance from the College of Insurance. He also holds Associate designations in Risk Management (ARM), Claims (AIC), and Marine Insurance Management (AMIM) from the Insurance Institute of America. Certifications include Lightning Safety Professional (CLSP), English XL VIT Tribometrist (CXLT), Safety Technician (CST), and Global Environment of Insurance (GEI).

---

[1] ESIS, Inc. (ESIS®) is a risk management services company of ACE USA. "ACE USA" refers to the insurance, reinsurance, and risk management companies comprising the U.S.-based operating division of the ACE Group of Companies, headed by ACE Limited.

Introduction (Statistics)

Each person takes an average of 18,000 steps a day, amounting to more than 6.5 million steps annually. This represents a tremendous exposure.

Falls in the workplace are the number one preventable loss type; in public places, falls are far and away the leading cause of injury. More than one million people suffer from a slip, trip, or fall injury each year, and more than 16,000 die as a result of falls, second only to automobiles as a cause of death (National Safety Council, 1999a). National Safety Council (NSC) statistics indicate that 25,000 slip and fall accidents occur daily in the U.S. The NSC estimates that compensation and medical costs associated with employee slip and fall accidents alone are approximately $70 billion.

Falls are estimated to cause 17% of occupational (work-related) injuries and 18% of public sector injuries (NSC); however, these figures are understated. Falls are notoriously underreported because accident rates are normally classified by injury type instead of cause of injury in workers' compensation and National Electronic Injury Surveillance System (NEISS) statistics. An estimated 300,000 disabling injuries occur each year in the U.S. workforce (National Institute for Occupational Safety and Health [NIOSH], 1998). According to the National Council on Compensation Insurance (NCCI), the average cost of a fall-related claim is almost $13,000, excluding indirect expenses, which can be several times this amount.

It should be no surprise that falls represent as much as half of all liability loss frequency and severity for insurance companies. Studies show that this category of loss ranges from 7% (for manufacturing) to 52% (for care providers), and higher still for restaurants. The situation is comparable overseas.

There is, understandably, great interest in methods to prevent falls. Contrary to popular belief, most slip/falls are not due to carelessness. Many options are available in the design and maintenance of facilities to reduce or eliminate the potential for slip/falls.

A review of slip/fall losses reveals that, in addition to contributory negligence of the accident victim, there is often something the property owner/management could have done to reduce the severity or prevent the incident. That "something" is often repairing a defect in the environment or a lack of management controls that contributed to the likelihood or severity of the event.

Changing Demographics

As baby boomers mature, the U.S. population is aging at a rapid rate. Individuals 55 years and older are the fastest-growing segment of the population, currently at around 31%. More than 6000 adults turn 65 every day. By the year 2030, the number of people over 65 is expected to double. By 2050, those over 65 will reach 80 million.

The increase in people age 85 and older is also substantial. By 2010, this segment will grow by 33%, from 4 million to 5.6 million.

In addition, the life expectancy of males and females continues to increase. By 2050, life expectancy for males is projected to go from 73 to 86, and from 79 to 92 for females.

These individuals are the country's workers and members of the general public. This older portion of U.S. citizens is most at risk for frequency and severity of slips and falls. Fall deaths increase with age, from a low of 40 (5 to 14 years old) to 11,900 (75 and over). As the number of older people increases, so does their potential for fall injuries. This increasing exposure to falls requires increased attention to controls associated with reducing and preventing fall injuries for workers and for the general public.

According to the Centers for Disease Control (CDC):

- One of every three people 65 years and older falls each year. This amounts to more than 11 million people.
- Older adults are hospitalized for fall-related injuries five times more often than they are for injuries from other causes. About 40% of all nursing facility admissions are the result of falls.
- Of those who fall, 20 to 30% suffer moderate to severe injury, which reduces mobility and independence and increases the risk of premature death.
- In 1994, the total direct cost of all fall injuries for people age 65 and older was $20.2 billion. By 2020, this figure is expected to reach $32.4 billion.

In addition, more than 10 million Americans have osteoporosis, and 18 million have low bone density. Both of these factors contribute to the severity of a fall.

More Statistics

Slips and falls are a multifaceted problem because they are a major cause of loss, not only to the general public (i.e., invitees, guests, patrons, customers, clients) but also to employees. Slips and falls are the second most frequent cause of worker injuries and personal injury incidents.

Note: These statistics should be considered low estimates. Falls are notoriously underreported because accident rates are normally classified by injury type instead of cause of injury in workers' compensation and NEISS statistics. Many accidents that are otherwise classified began with a slip, trip, or fall.

Deaths[1]

Due to Unintentional Injury

- Falls are second only to motor vehicle accidents as causes of death, accounting for 17,100 deaths in 1999 (a 6% increase from 1998, which was 8% higher than 1997). Deaths from falls have steadily increased:

[1] Unless otherwise attributed, excerpted from Injury Facts™, 1999 and 2000 Editions, National Safety Council, 2000.

13,450 (1994); 13,986 (1995); 14,986 (1996); 15,447 (1997); and 16,600 (1998). Falls also account for the second highest death rate (5.8 per 100,000 people). The death rate has not fallen during any year since 1986.

- Deaths from falls are fairly evenly divided by month, with a high of 1473 in January and a low of 1204 in June, indicating the small impact of weather-related incidents.

Due to Unintentional Public Injury (1999)

- Falls are the leading cause of unintentional public injury deaths, accounting for 6800 deaths (up 17% from 1998, which was 8% higher than 1997).

Due to Unintentional Home Injury (1998 and 1999)

- At 10,700, falls are the leading cause of unintentional injury deaths in the home (an increase of 9% from 1997).

Injuries*

Injury-Related Hospital Emergency Department Visits (1996, 1998)

- Accidental falls account for the most hospital visits (yes, even more than motor vehicle accidents) at 7.2 million, or almost 21% of all visits.
- Hospital visits due to stair/step falls alone have been steadily increasing throughout the past two decades, from a low of 695,968 (1980) to 989,826 (1998) (CPSC/NEISS).
- In 10 of the 12 age groups, falls account for the highest number of injuries requiring hospital treatment for six of them (0–4, 5–9, 35–44, 45–54, 55–64, and 65+). It is the second most frequent cause for the 10–14 age group, third for two other age groups (15–19 and 25–34), and fifth for ages 20–24.

Nonfatal Injury Costs (1995–1996)

- Falls on stairs/steps represent the highest cost of nonfatal injuries for 5 of the 12 age groups (falls on floors account for 3 more age groups). Falls are in the top 10 of all 12 age groups. Overall, falls from stairs/steps and floors rank number one and number two, respectively, accounting for 17% of nonfatal injury costs overall. The cost of stair-related injuries alone is estimated at $49.9 billion (Public Services Research Institute, from CPSC/NEISS data).

Nonfatal Occupational Injuries Involving Days Away from Work (1997)

- Same-level falls are the third most frequent type of nonfatal occupational injury, representing almost 14% of all losses (behind overexertion and contact with objects/equipment). Trade and services have the highest number of falls at 16.6% and 17.6%, respectively.
- Excluding motor vehicle accidents, the average cost of a worker fall ($12,470) is second only to burns ($12,792).

Other Statistics

- A 1985 study estimated that the total lifetime cost of injuries due to falls in the U.S. was $37.3 billion (Rice, D.P., Mackenzie, E.J. and Associates, 1989).
- Slips and falls is the leading category of kitchen injuries in restaurant/hospitality occupancies, accounting for 34% of all restaurant worker injury cases (Hedden, 1997).
- Falls account for 45% of all workers' compensation claim costs in restaurants (Liberty Mutual Insurance Company, 1995).
- A study by the Food Marketing Institute (FMI) found that 53% of all workers' compensation claims and public liability suits against supermarkets resulted from injuries sustained as a result of slip and fall accidents.

For more information on U.S. injury statistics, see the current edition of the NSC's Injury Facts publication (http://www.nsc.org).

Contents

1 Physical Evaluation

1.1 INTRODUCTION

In the U.S., there is substantial agreement regarding appropriate design dimensions of walkway surfaces and associated components. The most recognized codes in this area are the model building codes and the life safety code, all of which have long been in use and, consequently, have been well tested.

Physical evaluation related to slips and falls is one of the fundamentals to prevention. The importance of proper design cannot be overstated. Effective safety begins with good design. Ramps that are too steep, uneven steps, unmarked changes in levels, and missing handrails are major contributors to falls. Implementing effective management controls will have a limited impact if good design is not in place.

1.2 EXPECTATION

When walkway surface conditions encountered are different from what is expected, the potential for an accident increases.

"Expectation" is the underlying principle of effective slip/trip/fall evaluations. For example, if we are aware of the ice or water ahead, we can either attempt to avoid it *or* adjust our gait (i.e., the way we walk) to compensate for the differing surface. We will slow down, take smaller steps, and walk flatter. These subtle adjustments we make in the way we walk are likely to allow us to safely cross the hazardous area.

If we are *not* aware of the ice, however, we can neither avoid nor compensate our gait for the hazard. Numerous studies have consistently shown that individuals can cross a slippery area if they are aware of the condition.

Thus, the most effective option for preventing falls is to either eliminate unexpected conditions that constitute slip and fall hazards, or (less desirable) assure that pedestrians receive clear notice of the presence of such conditions so they can be adequately prepared to deal with them.

1.3 DISTRACTIONS

It is important to recognize the impact that distractions can have on pedestrians. Avoid extensive signage and eye-catching images and designs in areas where pedestrians need to be aware of where they are walking. Areas of great concern are stairs, escalators, at floor surface transitions, a change in levels (short flights of three steps or less), entryways where contaminants and moisture can accumulate, and congested areas.

1.4 LEVEL WALKWAY SURFACES

Based on several references, including the Americans with Disabilities Act (ADA) and American Society of Testing and Materials (ASTM) F-1637 (see "Reference Standards" at the end of this chapter), a trip hazard is defined as a change in elevation in a walkway that is not a proper ramp or stairway, with a vertical face $^{1}/_{4}$ in. or higher, or a change in elevation of more than $^{1}/_{4}$ in. with an inclined face steeper than two horizontal on one vertical. Stride studies have shown that subjects with low-heeled shoes clear the ground by a mere $^{1}/_{4}$ in., and less by those with higher-heeled shoes. Thus, a seemingly minimal but sudden increase in the walkway surface can readily result in a trip.

The following paragraphs outline some guidelines in evaluating the degree of hazard of level walking surfaces.

1.4.1 SIDEWALKS

Identify surfaces with cracks, potholes, or other conditions that could contribute to a fall. Settlement of asphalt and concrete surfaces can often create these conditions, as can concrete spalling. Walkway surfaces should be free of debris and other slippery material (e.g., gravel, mud, sand, food spills), and other similar materials.

In practice, cracks in sidewalks are not normally a problem if the slabs are not heaved; but a vertical surface discontinuity of $^{1}/_{4}$ in. can trip many pedestrians because it may be unexpected.

A simple and practical way to determine such small differences is to use pennies. With a thickness of $^{1}/_{16}$ in., stacking two pennies gives you a rule for $^{1}/_{8}$ in., and four pennies a rule for $^{1}/_{4}$ in. (see Figure 1.1, Figure 1.2, and Figure 1.3).

1.4.2 CURBING

The standard height for curbs in the U.S. is 6 in. Curbs of different heights due to design or settling can create an unexpected condition for pedestrians, increasing the potential for falls.

Curbing leading to sidewalks and entrances should be painted a contrasting color. Unless curbs are painted yellow to denote "no parking" areas, good choices are white or red (Figure 1.4).

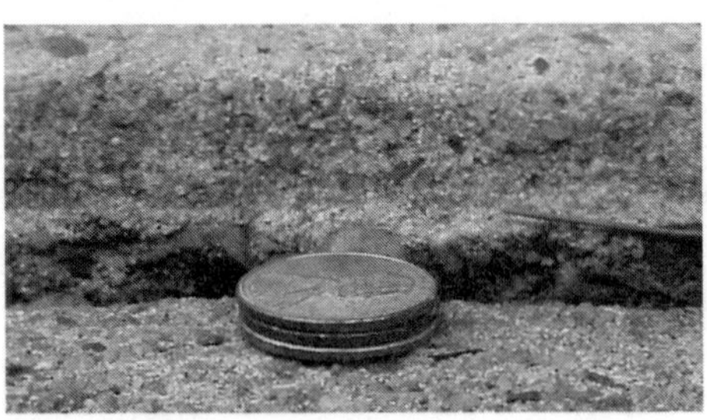

FIGURE 1.1 Measuring small differences with pennies.

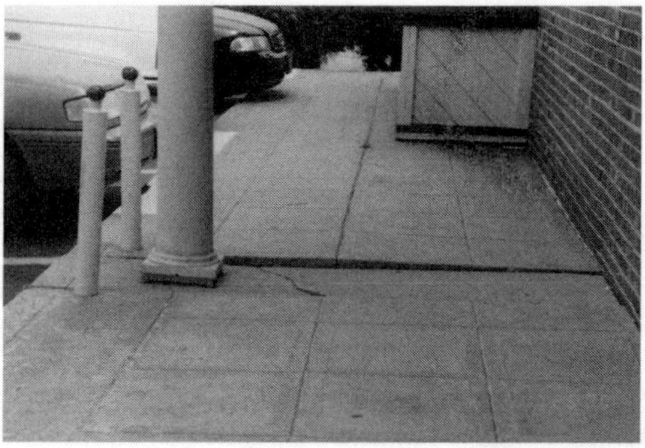

FIGURE 1.2 The "Before" picture — It is not difficult to see the tripping hazard in this picture, spanning the entire walkway area. Probably due to settling, the difference in level ranges from about $^{1}/_{4}$ in. to almost 2 in. (Photograph courtesy of K. Vidal.)

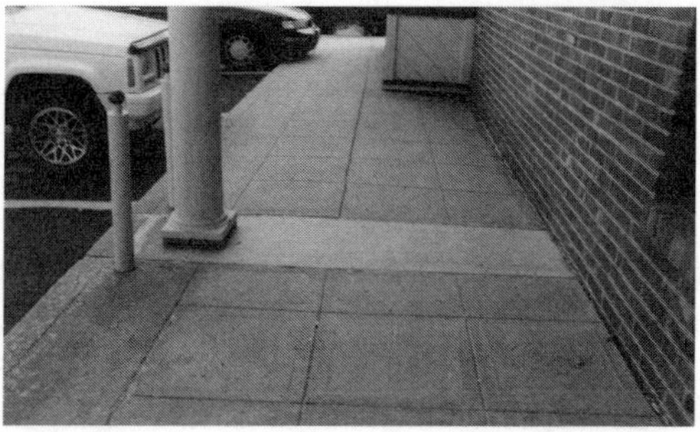

FIGURE 1.3 The "After" picture — a good job of correcting the problem. (Photograph courtesy of K. Vidal.)

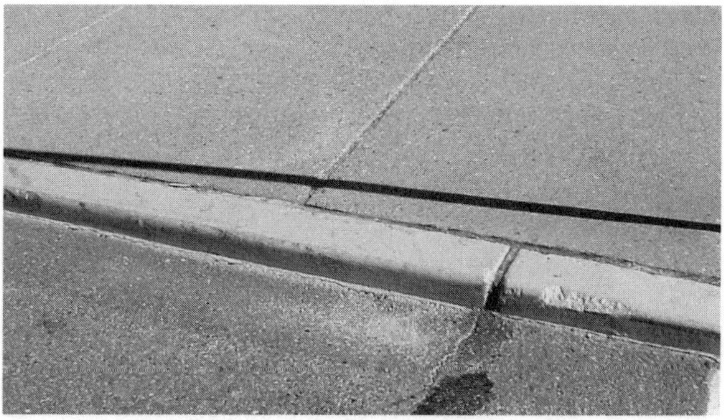

FIGURE 1.4 The curb is certainly well marked because it is painted a bright yellow; however, the height of the curb is substantially lower than the expected 6-in. standard.

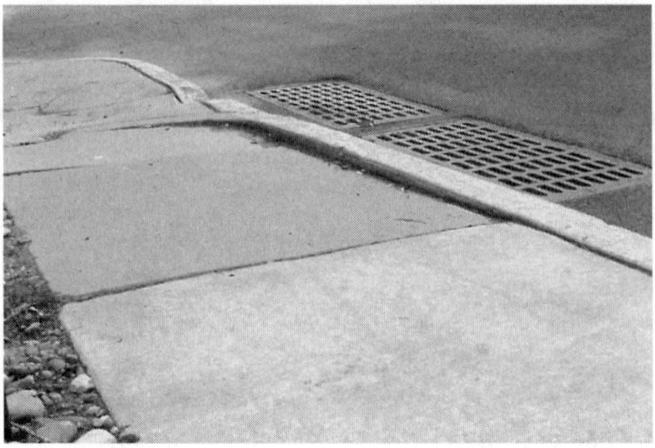

FIGURE 1.5 Aside from the cracking and unevenness of the sidewalk, the major issue is the extreme settlement of the sidewalk. The curbing (a separate piece) remains as it was constructed, which presents a significant trip hazard. The addition of drainage grates, which can be slippery and can accumulate water/ice when blocked, makes it a high-potential area for falls.

Curbing is constructed in two ways. The first is as a separate extruded piece of concrete, independent of the sidewalk. Depending on soil conditions and weather, this construction carries a high risk of settling and results in uneven surfaces between the curb and the sidewalk. Extruded curbing is usually evident by the concrete gutter that extends out into the roadway. The second type is more stable, in which the curbing and sidewalk are a single piece of concrete, thus minimizing the potential for gaps and unevenness between them as settlement and weather take their tolls (see Figure 1.5 and Figure 1.6).

1.4.3 Curb CutOuts

The primary purpose of curb cutouts is to provide a means of making exterior walkways accessible to persons with disabilities, particularly those in wheelchairs; however, there are proper and improper designs for curb cutouts. If not done properly, cutouts can become substantial trip and fall hazards.

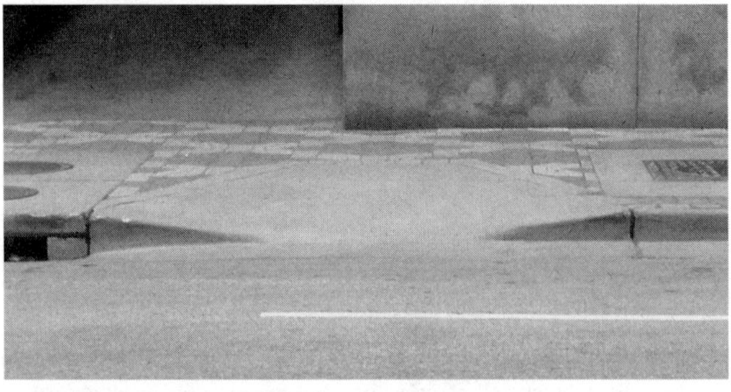

FIGURE 1.6 Although not well marked, the overall design with flared sides is a good one.

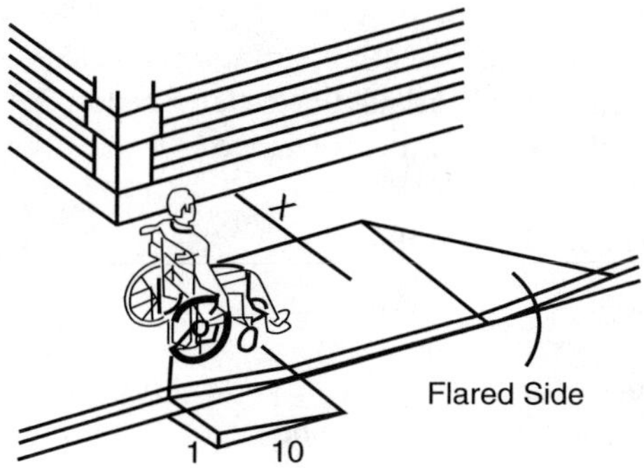

FIGURE 1.7 Where the curb ramp is completely contained within a planting strip or other nonwalking surface, so that pedestrians would not normally cross the sides, the curb ramp sides can have steep sides including vertical returned curbs (from ADA Figure 12B). This figure shows a typical curb ramp (cut into a walkway perpendicular to the curb face) with flared sides having a maximum slope of 1:10. The landing at the top, measured from the top of the ramp to the edge of the walkway or closest obstruction is denoted as "x." If x (the landing depth at the top of a curb ramp) is less than 48 in., then the slope of the flared side shall not exceed 1:12 (from ADA Figure 12A).

Whenever possible, however, building grading should be designed to avoid the need for cutouts.

The American National Standards Institute (ANSI) A117.1 standard, Accessible and Usable Buildings and Facilities from the International Code Council, provides curb cutout design specifications in section 406 (Figure 1.7 and Figure 1.8).

- Similar to all ramps, curb cutouts should not exceed 1:12.
- Do not permit curb edging to extend above the cutout slope. Instead, the ramp should have flared sides (a maximum slope of 1:10). If edging is present, a landscaped area or other barrier should be provided to prevent individuals from crossing over the raised curb area.

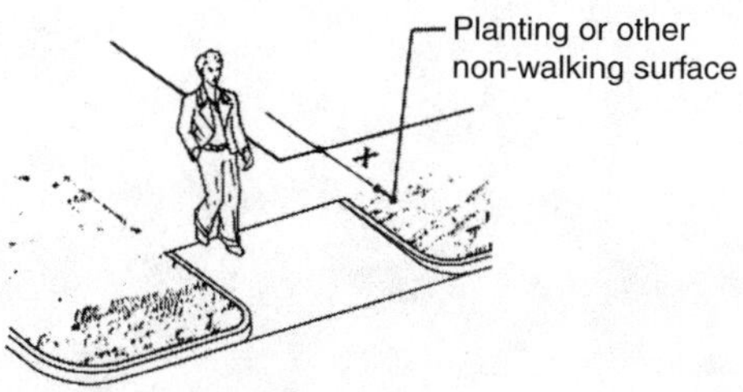

FIGURE 1.8 Where the curb ramp is completely contained within a planting strip or other nonwalking surface, so that pedestrians would not normally cross the sides, the curb ramp sides can have steep sides including vertical returned curbs (from ADA Figure 12B). This figure shows a typical curb ramp (cut into a walkway perpendicular to the curb face) with flared sides having a maximum slope of 1:10. The landing at the top, measured from the top of the ramp to the edge of the walkway or closest obstruction is denoted as "x." If x (the landing depth at the top of a curb ramp) is less than 48 in., then the slope of the flared side shall not exceed 1:12. (from ADA Figure 12A).

If cutout ramps are painted, paint with a slip resistant paint. This usually means grit has been added to the mix, creating surface roughness. Although there is no requirement that curb ramps be marked, the issue of pedestrian expectation suggests there should be a visual cue indicating a change in walkway surfaces.

1.4.4 Other Walkway Impediments

1.4.4.1 Access Covers

Access covers take many forms and may be present for many reasons. Usually, they are to provide access to a valve located underground for a utility (e.g., water, gas, cable). Junction boxes and any similar access covers (such as gas and sewers) in parking lots or in walkway paths should be designed to be flush with the surface (Figure 1.9).

No practical reason exists to have a protrusion above the surface. Optimally, underground lines should be located so that access is not required in an obvious pedestrian path.

1.4.4.2 Drainage Grates

Commonly encountered in parking lots, drain gratings often have excessively wide openings, as wide as 3 in. Some are designed with convex covers, making them even more hazardous to traverse, especially for people wearing high-heeled shoes and similar footwear (Figure 1.10).

Drain grates are usually recessed to some degree to permit the channeling of water from other areas to the drain. Some are excessively graded, however, and settlement of the surface makes that slope even more extreme.

Most drainage grates tend to fade visually into parking lots since they are as black as the asphalt. For purposes of pedestrian safety, however, consideration should

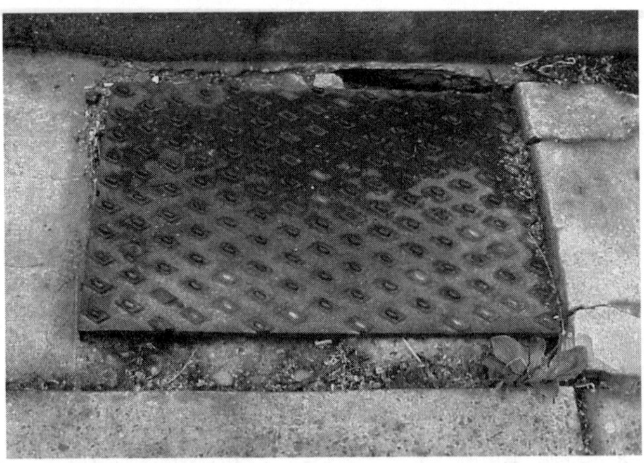

FIGURE 1.9 The condition, stability, and protrusions of this access cover clearly make it a poor example.

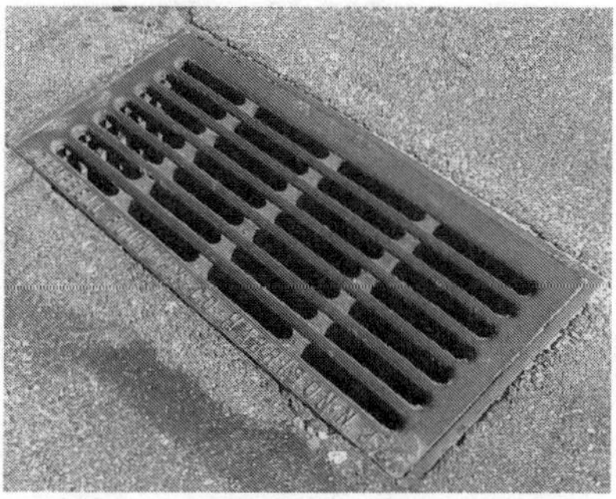

FIGURE 1.10 A typical drainage grate found in parking lots. Note the large openings and uneven surface.

be given to painting drainage grates a bright color like yellow. This will serve to increase the awareness of pedestrians to an increased walking hazard. It can also be of benefit to vehicles traversing the area.

Optimally, when designing drainage, locate grates away from natural pedestrian paths. ASTM F-1637 recommends that such grates should have openings no wider than $^1/_2$ in. in the predominant direction of travel.

1.4.4.3 Posts

In most cases, posts are unnecessary evils. They can cause damage while protecting little of consequence. Damaged posts become greater hazards to pedestrians, especially when broken off close to the ground and with sharp edges. In many cases, posts remain long after the object they were intended to protect has been removed (Figure 1.11).

If posts are used, they must be substantial enough to withstand the punishment anticipated. They should also be painted a high-contrast color so they will be readily seen.

1.4.4.4 Bicycle Racks

Bicycle racks should be placed away from vehicle and pedestrian traffic, and arranged such that their walkway-level supports do not impinge on the walkway path.

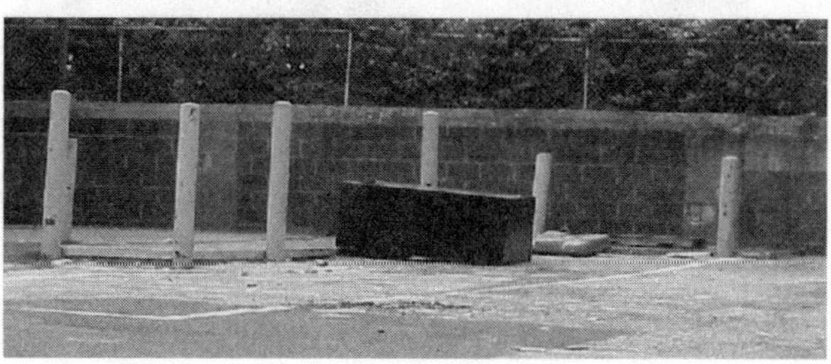

FIGURE 1.11 This "pole farm" consists of seven poles in various states of disrepair, which protect nothing.

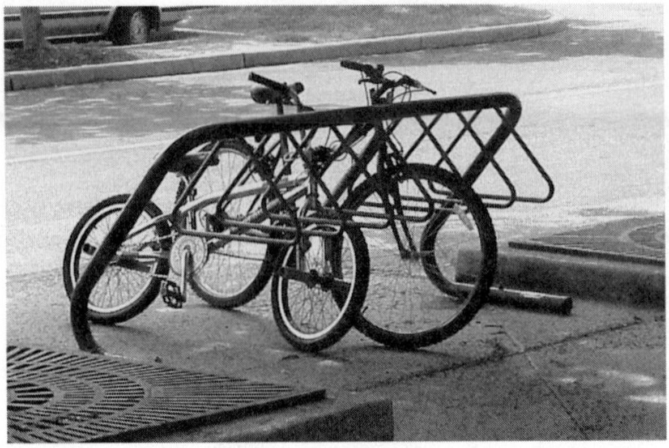

FIGURE 1.12 A typical bike rack arrangement. Although this rack is set inside an untraveled area, bikes placed here do protrude out into the walkway.

It is also helpful if they are painted a bright color such as yellow or white (Figure 1.12).

1.4.4.5 Planters, Trash Receptacles, and Similar Furnishings

The configuration, visibility, and location of these furnishings affect their potential for contributing to falls (Figure 1.13).

Planters with sharp bases, or those that extend out into the walkway present a greater risk, as do other protrusions that are designed to fade into the scenery.

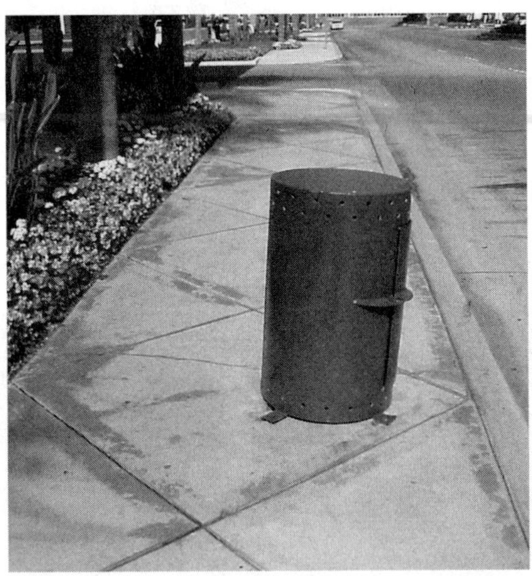

FIGURE 1.13 This blockage was moved into the walkway path to cover a hole in the sidewalk — a modest improvement at best.

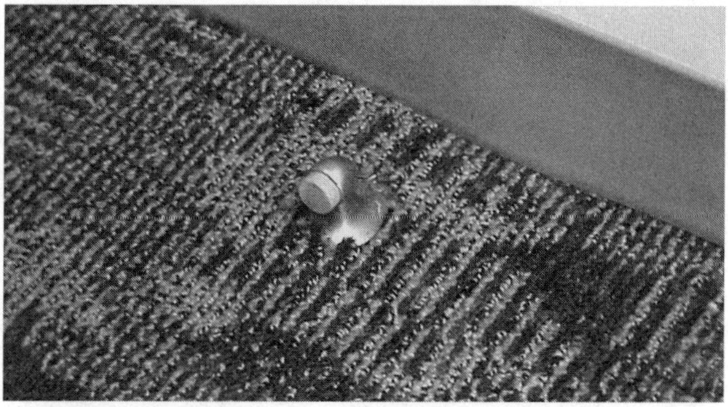

FIGURE 1.14 A well-camouflaged doorstop.

1.4.4.6 Architectural Designs

Architectural designs can create fall hazards because they are not easily seen and because they are otherwise unexpected by the pedestrian.

1.4.4.7 Sprinkler Heads, Doorstops, and Other Small Trip Hazards

The harder they are to see, the greater the hazard they pose. The cost-benefits of small trip hazards need to be carefully evaluated. Then, placement and marking should be considered if necessary (Figure 1.14).

1.4.4.8 Temporary Fixes

All too common are temporary fixes — obstructions placed in the walkway for a variety of reasons. Some are to protect an opening from water infiltration or damage. Others are a misguided effort to prevent pedestrian falls. Such half-hearted repairs often remain in place for a period substantially longer than originally intended, and frequently create or increase the hazard (Figure 1.15).

1.5 LEVEL WALKWAY SURFACES AND WATER

The facility should be designed and maintained to prohibit (or at least minimize) the accumulation of water in walkway areas and around building areas.

Aside from the hazard posed by the water alone, cold weather increases the likelihood that such accumulations will turn into ice, thereby compounding the hazard (Figure 1.16).

A variety of conditions can contribute to water accumulation:

- Inadequate grading of land away from the building
- Depressions, holes, and other concave areas as a result of settling
- Inadequate storm drainage capability or blocked drains
- Inadequate gutter capability, or drainage of gutter into a pedestrian path

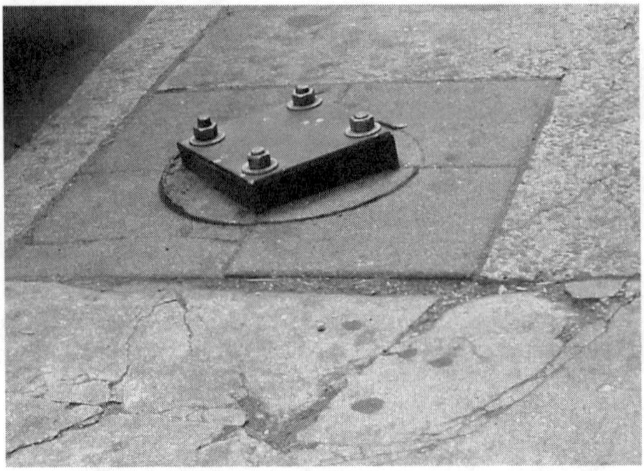

FIGURE 1.15 A substantial protrusion, intended to protect an opening left by removal of a light pole.

- Air-conditioning system condensation
- Lawn sprinkler overspray

1.6 PARKING AREAS

Similar to sidewalks and other level walkway surfaces, cracks, holes, and other blemishes need to be regularly identified and corrected. The guidelines are the same, in practice $^1/_8$ in. or $^1/_4$ in. In addition to the issues related to level walking surfaces mentioned previously, however, parking areas have additional design needs. They are a challenge to maintain primarily because they are subject to heavy, concentrated foot and vehicle traffic during operating hours.

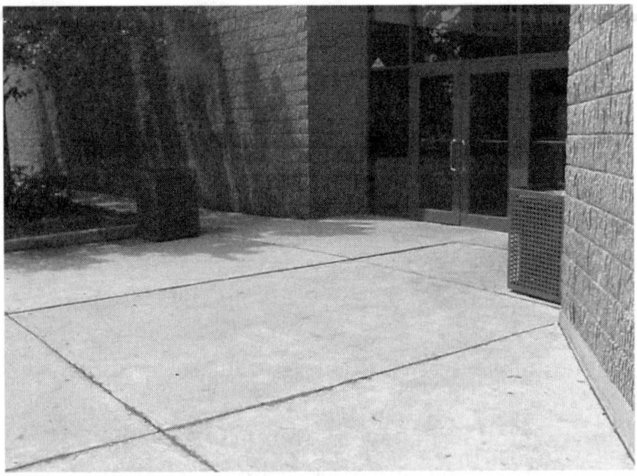

FIGURE 1.16 A good example of grading away from the entrance area, thus avoiding water accumulation.

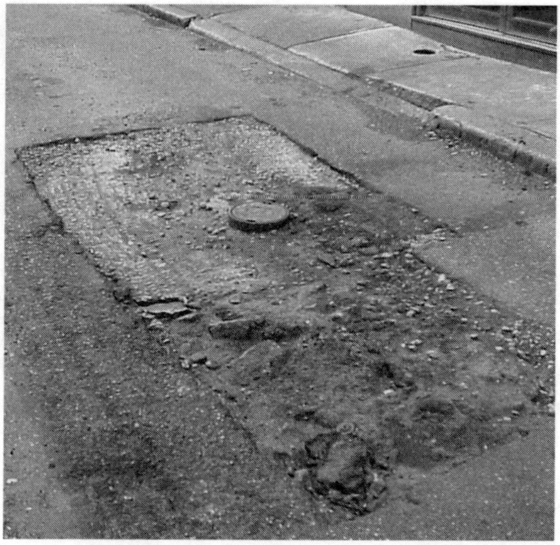

FIGURE 1.17 An extreme example of conditions that can develop in parking lots.

Weather, vehicle accidents, and plows can all cause damage. Left unrepaired, these kinds of problems become more and more severe, increasing the potential for injury to pedestrians. In addition to assuring asphalt surfaces are in good condition, making sure exterior lighting is maintained can reduce risk potential (Figure 1.17).

1.6.1 Tire Stops

Parking lots can and should be designed without tire stops. Tire stops require maintenance, are often damaged by snowplows and other vehicles, and are a common tripping hazard (Figure 1.18).

In some instances, the presence of tire stops in newly designed parking lots can be considered poor design (Figure 1.19).

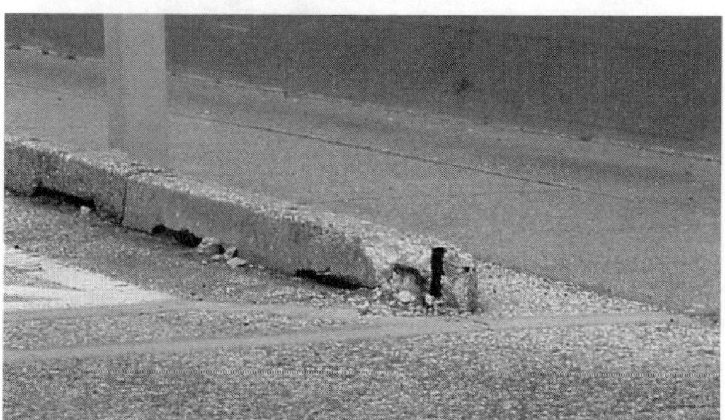

FIGURE 1.18 Tire stops are subject to substantial punishment and must be inspected and maintained.

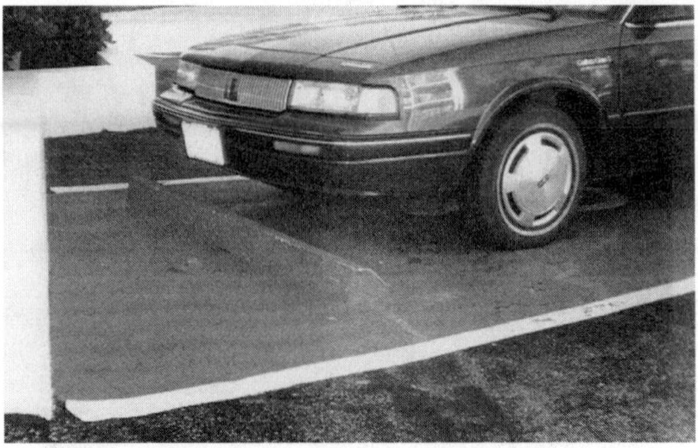

FIGURE 1.19 This tire stop is well marked, strongly contrasting with its surroundings, and is in good repair. Constructed of recycled rubber, it is also more durable and resilient. (Photograph courtesy of K. Vidal.)

Where tire stops are present, several precautions should be observed (Figure 1.20):

- The maximum height should be $6^1/_2$ in. with at least 3 ft between wheel stops.
- To minimize the tripping hazard, tire stops should not protrude beyond the width of tires.
- Tire stops should be well marked with a contrasting color so they do not blend in with the parking lot, especially at night.
- Tire stops of railroad tie construction deteriorate much more quickly, presenting an increased hazard.
- Reinforcing bar and other methods of securement should not extend beyond the tire stop itself.

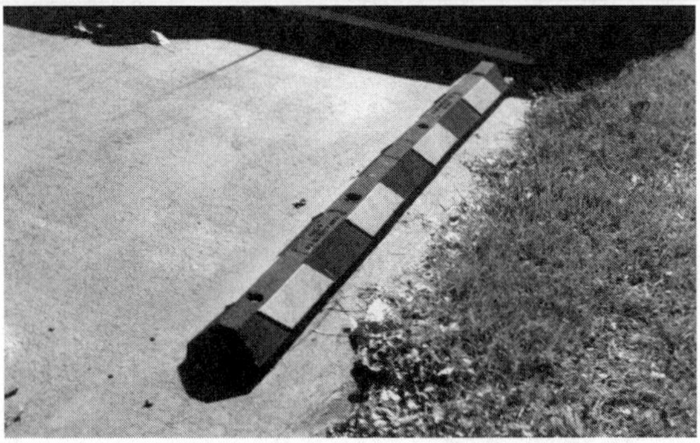

FIGURE 1.20 This tire stop has been cleverly disguised to blend in with the floor surface, effectively making it invisible to many pedestrians. Although it is not a major concern when a vehicle is parked here (as long as the driver can see it while parking), the tire stop presents a serious trip hazard when the spot is unoccupied. (Photograph courtesy of K. Vidal.)

1.6.2 Speed Bumps

Although national and professional standards have been established for components of public transportation roadway systems, no standards have been issued from an adoptive government body or agency for "traffic calming" devices. Two nationally accepted transportation standards, the *Manual on Uniform Traffic Control Devices for Streets and Highways* (MUTCD), established by the U.S. Federal Highway Administration, and *A Policy of Geometric Design of Highways and Streets,* produced by the American Association of State Highway and Transportation Officials, are silent as to required design features or placement of traffic calming devices.

After automobiles were invented at the turn of the 20th century, and their use became abundant and common, local governments were immediately confronted with how to control their speeds. As such, the traffic calming issue of today is by far nothing new. The actual idea of using physical barriers began early on with the installation of speed bumps on public streets. Speed "bumps" are typically found in parking lots. They differ greatly from the speed "humps" encountered on some public roadways, which are much longer and more gradual than speed bumps (see Figure 1.21 and Figure 1.22).

A properly designed speed hump should not affect traffic flow and comfort much, unless the vehicles are traveling above 30 mph or so, or are very heavily loaded. Speed humps generally are 12 ft to 22 ft wide, and are generally 3 or 4 in. in height, whereas older speed bumps were only 3 to 36 in. wide and 3 to 6 in. high (Klik and Faghri, 1993); however, their public use was short-lived.

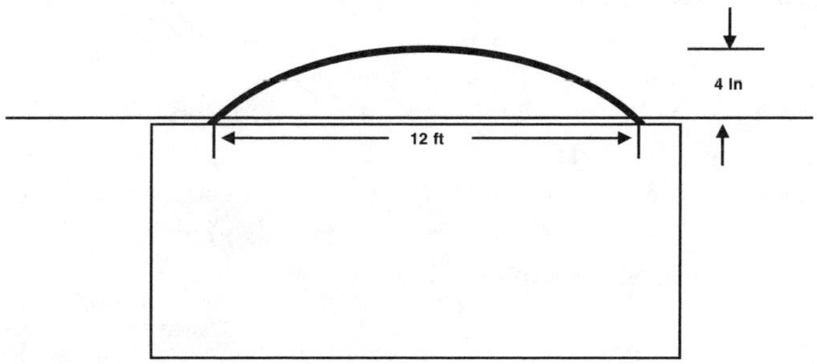

FIGURE 1.21 Speed hump.

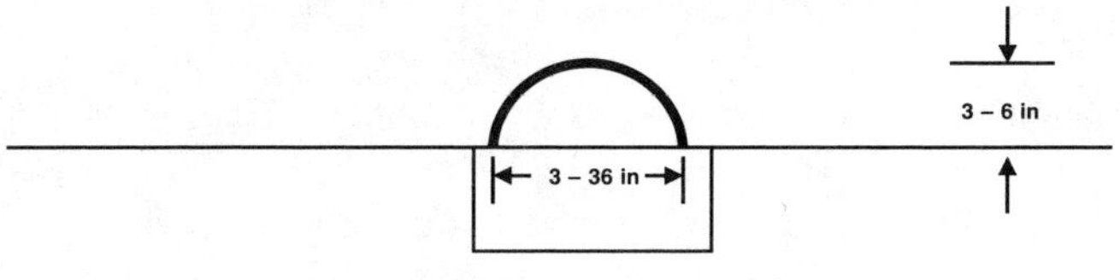

FIGURE 1.22 Speed bump.

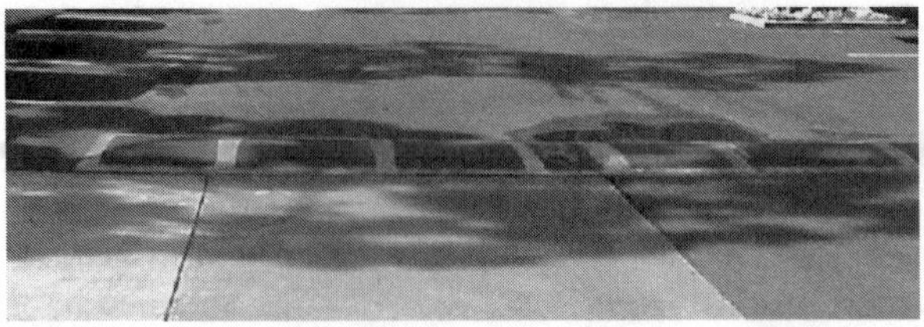

FIGURE 1.23 Although it is fairly well marked with yellow stripes, this speed bump also spans a frequent and natural pedestrian walkway area.

Similar to tire stops, speed bumps are usually unnecessary in properly designed parking lots. The layout of the lot should make it impractical to drive at high speeds. Speed bumps can cause damage to vehicles and can be damaged by snowplows. Unrealized by most drivers, heavy automobiles can more smoothly pass over them at 35 mph than at slower speeds (Figure 1.23).

Usually constructed from asphalt, severe weather can accelerate the deterioration of speed bumps.

Speed bumps can pose a tripping hazard, and should be located away from natural pedestrian paths, and entrance and exit areas.

Where speed bumps exist, they should be painted white or yellow to contrast with the parking lot. ANSI Z-535.1 Safety Color Coding provides specific guidance on such marking. It is advisable to provide signage indicating the presence of speed bumps.

The *Manual on Uniform Traffic Control Devices for Streets and Highways,* 2001 (U.S. Federal Highway Administration) provides specifications regarding marking and signage, but not design or dimensional criteria. This publication can be obtained in PDF format at http://mutcd.fhwa.dot.gov/.

ASTM F-1637 *Practice for Safe Walking Surfaces* (1995), sections 7 ("Speed Bumps"), and 4.2 ("Walkway Changes in Level") by reference indicates that speed bumps should be avoided in design. If they are used, they should not be in pedestrian paths. If they are in pedestrian paths, they should be marked according to ANSI Z535.1 with slip-resistant paint; caution signs are also recommended.

Other publications on the topic include:

- *Guidelines for the Design and Application of Speed Humps,* Institute of Transportation Engineers (ITE) Task Force TENC-5TF-01 Staff, published by the ITE (1993).
- *A Policy on Geometric Design of Highways and Streets 2001* — This fourth edition "Green Book" contains the latest design practices in universal use as the standard of highway geometric design.

More information is also available at http://www.digitalthreads.com/utarpt/utarpt5.html.

According to the MUTCD, Figure 1.24 and Figure 1.25 illustrate the requirements for signage relating to speed bumps and humps.

According to the MUTCD, Figure 1.26 presents the two common options for marking of speed humps:

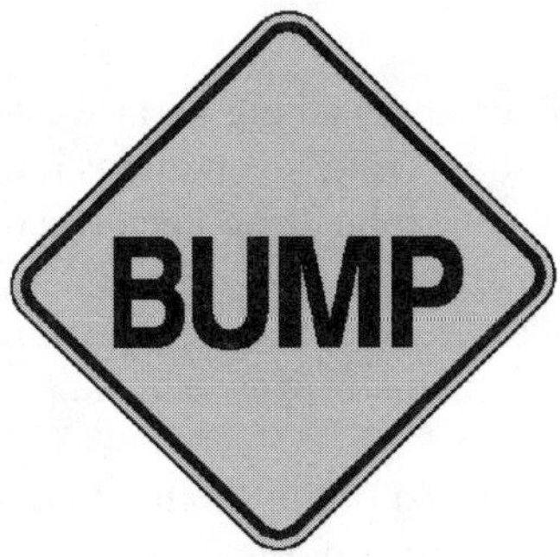

FIGURE 1.24 Bump Sign: Used to give warning of a sharp rise in the profile of the road. This sign may be supplemented with an Advisory Speed plaque.

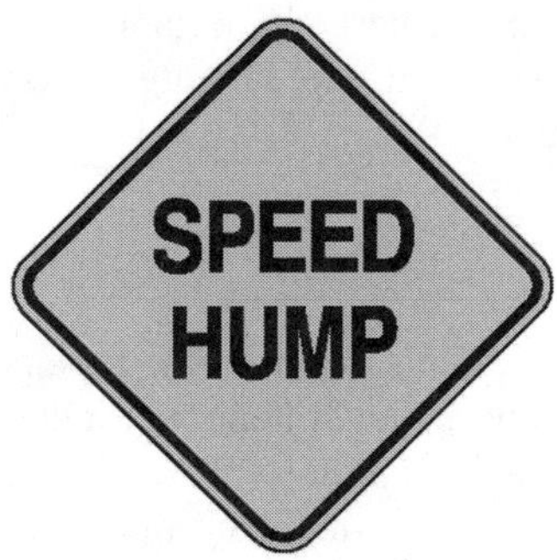

FIGURE 1.25 Speed Hump Sign: Used to give warning of a vertical deflection in the roadway that is designed to limit the speed of traffic. This sign should be supplemented by an Advisory Speed plaque.

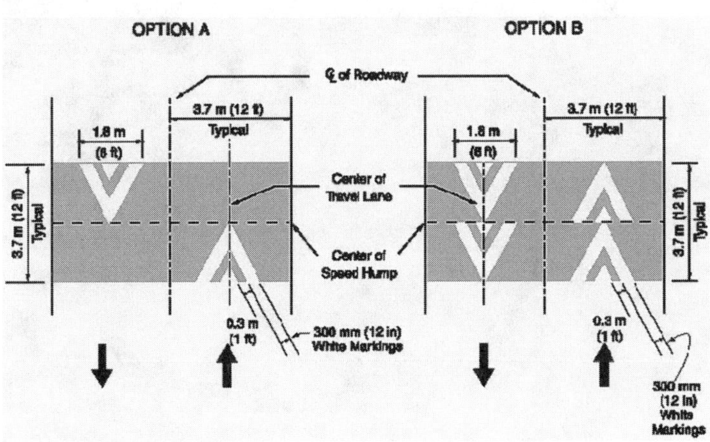

FIGURE 1.26 MUTCD speed bump marking options.

1.7 CHANGES IN LEVELS

Unmarked or unidentified floor and walking surface level changes are a source of severe fall claims. This exposure includes conditions ranging from recessed seating to a subtle height change from one room to another, to a quick step down just outside of a door.

In general, building codes are silent on requirements for short flight designs; however, there is some agreement on designs to avoid an unexpected change in level from a doorway.

The rule of thumb (also spelled out in the International Building Code) is that the landing on both sides of a doorway (i.e., the inside and outside) should be as long as the doorway is wide, and at least 44 in. in the direction of travel (Figure 1.27).

Where practical, short flights should be converted to a qualifying ramp. Otherwise, effective controls can include the use of contrasting colors, special lighting features, and warning signs. The goal is to provide visual cues to make the pedestrian aware of a change. This is particularly important for short flight step changes in which, from the perspective of the approaching pedestrian, the change is barely noticeable or not noticeable at all.

1.8 STAIRS

Seventy percent of all stair accidents occur on the top and bottom three steps. Maintenance and code variations are the main items to evaluate for stairs and landings.

National Fire Protection Association (NFPA) 101, the Life Safety Code (NFPA, 2000), is a consensus standard — a national voluntary standard that has, in many jurisdictions, become law in some form. As such, compliance (or lack of compliance) with this standard has a strong impact in the courts. As important, the life safety code specifications are tried-and-true guidelines for safe stairs (Figure 1.28).

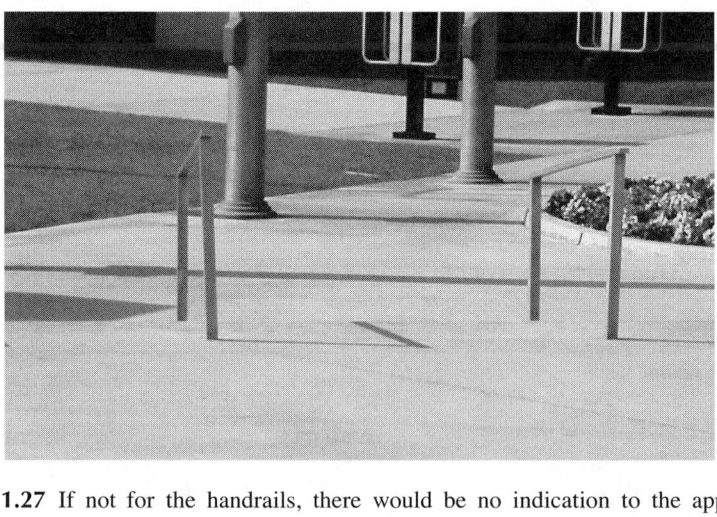

FIGURE 1.27 If not for the handrails, there would be no indication to the approaching pedestrian that a change in level was present.

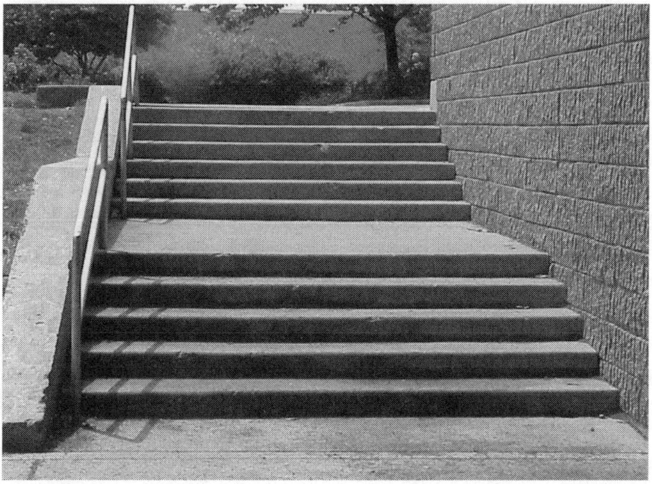

FIGURE 1.28 Although dimensionally sound, the condition of the stair nosings is questionable, and the single railing is inadequate.

1.8.1 Stair Design

- The rise angle of stairways should be between 30 and 35 degrees of slope.
- Stair riser height should be from 7 in. or 7 1/2 in. (existing) or 8 in. (new), with no deviation between adjacent risers exceeding 3/16 in.
- Stair riser height should deviate no more than 3/8 in. over the entire flight.
- Stair tread depth should range from 9 in. or 10 in. (existing) or 11 in. (new), with no deviation exceeding 3/16 in.
- Stair width should be at least 44 in. clear width, 36 in. if serving fewer than 50 occupants.
- Nosing should not protrude out more than 1 1/2 in. and should be beveled to reduce trip potential. The surface of treads should be of nonslip material.

(See Figure 1.29 and Figure 1.30.) Stairs should be uniform in tread width and riser height. The human body is an amazingly precise machine. It can detect subtle changes in elevation and distance. Thus, a change in riser height as small as 3/16 in. can disrupt a person's gait or walking rhythm (cadence) and significantly increases the potential for a fall.

1.8.2 Stair Landings

Per NFPA 101 7.2.2.3.2, stairs are required to have landings at door openings. Landings should have a consistent width; the width should be at least that of the stairs to which it is connected.

As specified by most building codes, and by NFPA for new construction, stair landings should be at least as long as the width of the stair. Thus, if the stair width is 36 in., the length (in the direction of travel) should be at least 36 in. This provision is made in order to avoid a door that opens directly onto the stair tread.

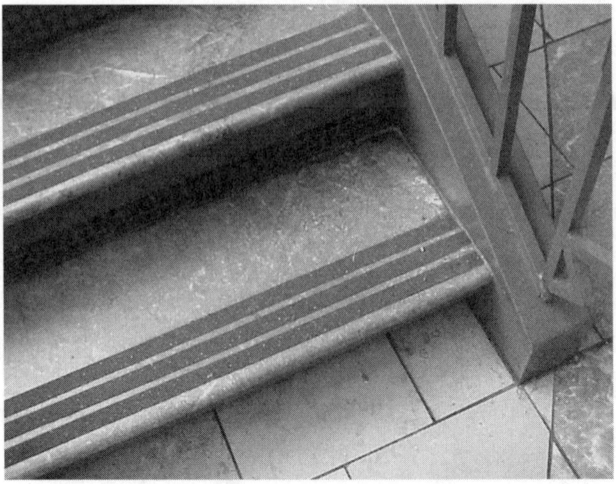

FIGURE 1.29 Good design and condition.

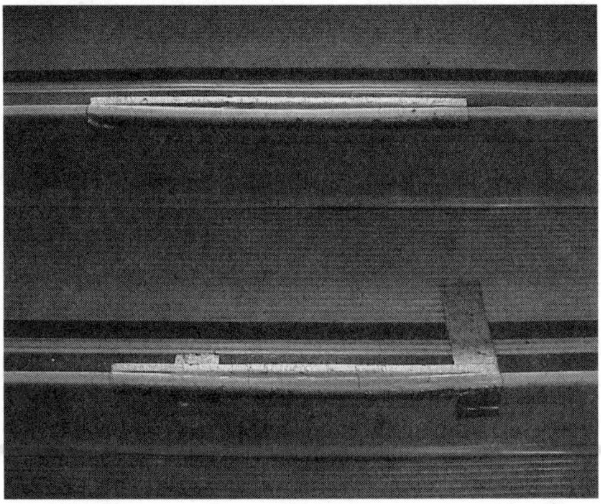

FIGURE 1.30 Poor condition and repair attempt.

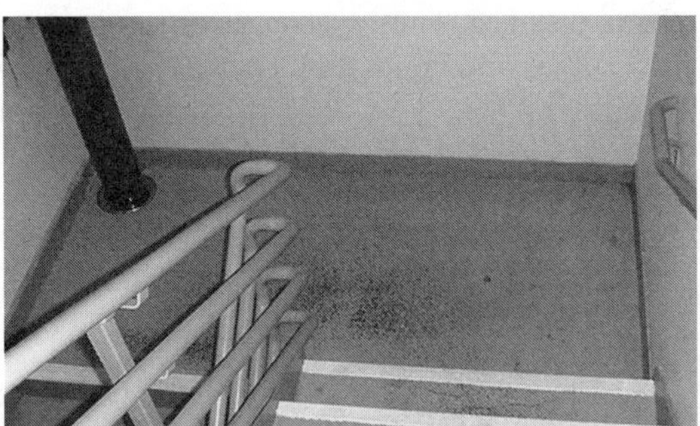

FIGURE 1.31 A suitable dimensional design for a stair landing.

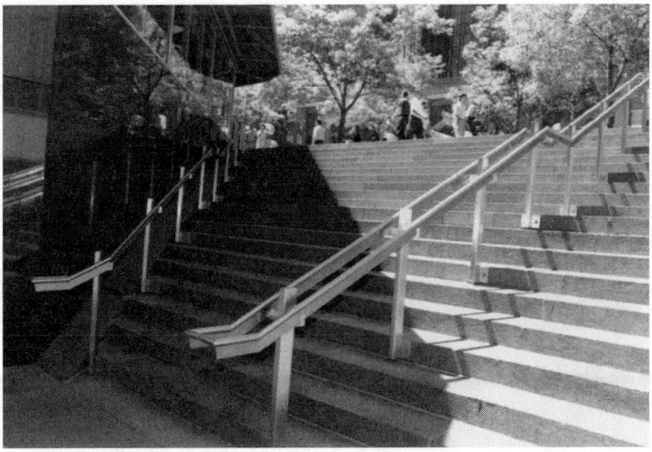

FIGURE 1.32 Although the railings are well spaced at the base of the stairs, they become progressively less useful higher on the flight. They are also not "graspable." (Photograph courtesy of K. Vidal.)

Landings need to be kept clear of storage or any other materials at all times in order to minimize congestion and ensure that adequate space passage is available (Figure 1.31).

1.9 HANDRAILS

Per NFPA 101 7.2.2.4, handrails should be accessible within 30 in. (for new buildings) and 44 in. (for existing buildings) of all portions of stair width. This is to ensure that, even if standing in the most remote part of the stair (farthest away from a handrail), a person should be able to reach out and grasp a handrail (Figure 1.32).

If a handrail is on only one side of the stair, a person should be able to reach it while standing against the other side of the stair. If handrails are on both sides, a person should be able to stand in the center of the stairs and reach either handrail.

Handrails should be between 34 in. and 38 in. in height, based on anthropometric data on the height of most adults. This ensures that the handrail will be above the center of gravity, reducing the potential for someone to lean and fall over a handrail.

1.9.1 Graspability

Unfortunately, designers often see handrails as aesthetic elements of building construction instead of essential safety features. Thus, handrails are frequently too wide or otherwise poorly designed for building occupants to grasp (see Figure 1.33 and Figure 1.34).

Handrails must have a diameter of $1\frac{1}{4}$ in. to $1\frac{1}{2}$ in. and must be positioned at least $1\frac{1}{2}$ in. from the wall. This specification considers the varied hand size of men and women, as well as the reduced hand strength of older individuals, and is intended to assure that the handrail can be gripped properly.

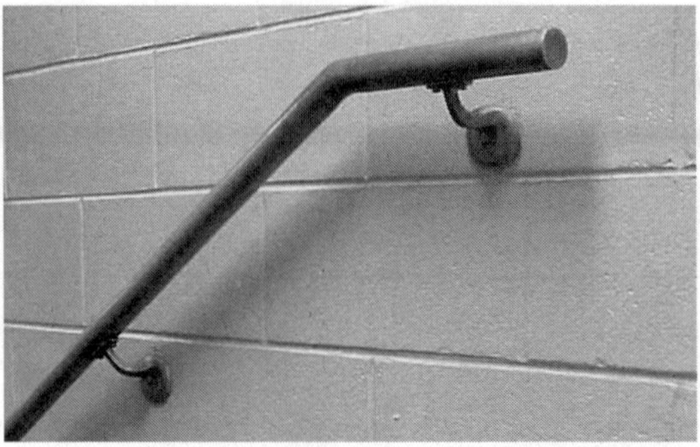

FIGURE 1.33 A graspable handrail extending beyond the stair — a good design.

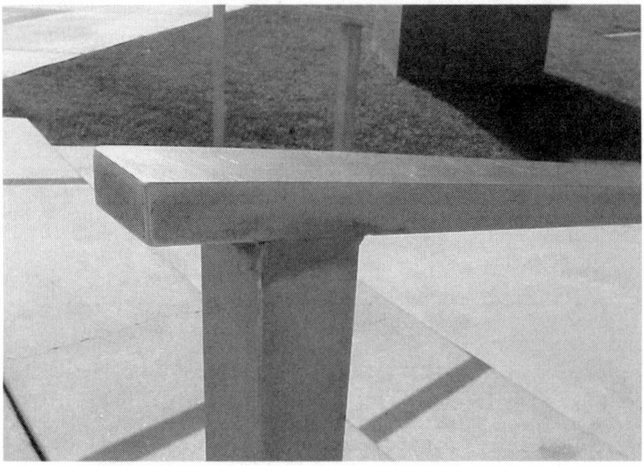

FIGURE 1.34 A squared cross section of handrail — difficult to grasp.

Handrails should extend beyond the stairway so the user can maintain a hold on it while taking the last step to the floor.

1.9.2 Supports

Handrail supports should be vertical, not horizontal. In essence, horizontal rails constitute a ladder to young children, who have been known to climb it and fall over the other side (Figure 1.35).

Handrail supports should not permit the passage of a 4-in. sphere — this precludes children from getting their heads stuck between the rails.

1.10 GUARDS (OR GUARDRAILS)

Per NFPA 101 7.2.2.4.6, in order to reduce the potential for falls, guards should be provided where stairs are at a height 30 in. or more above the floor level.

Located above handrails, guards should be at least 42 in. in height (Figure 1.36).

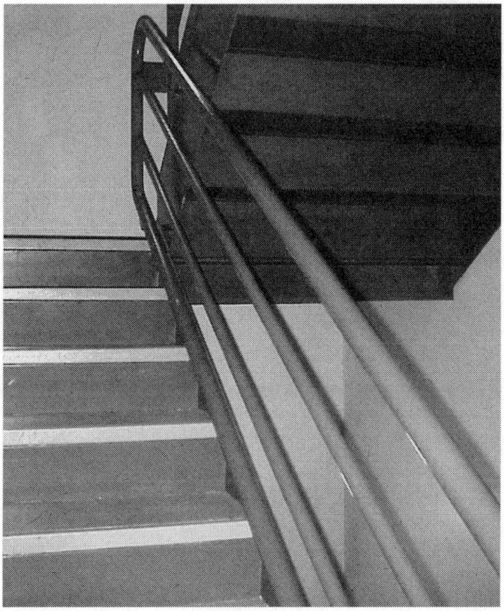

FIGURE 1.35 Horizontal supports can be unintentionally used for climbing.

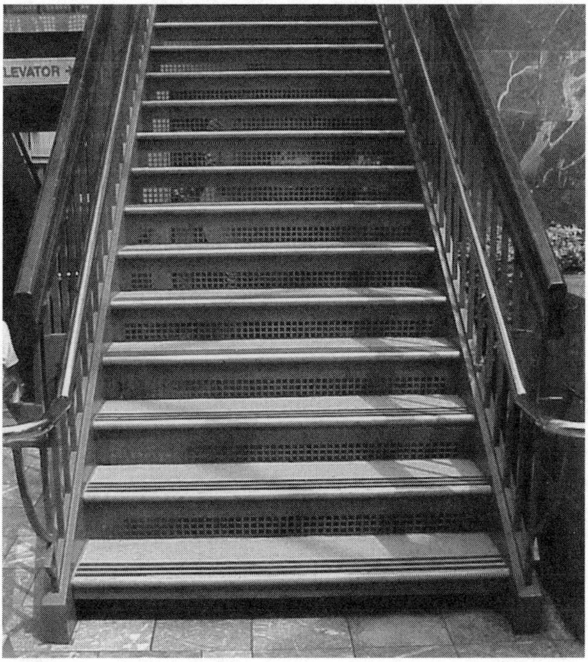

FIGURE 1.36 Handrails with guardrails above.

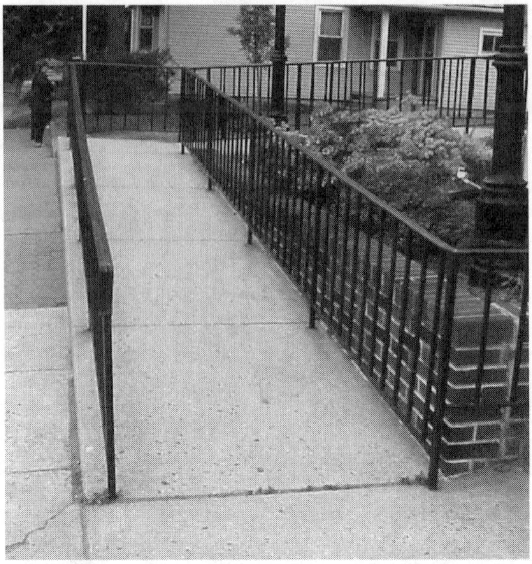

FIGURE 1.37 A good ramp design, retrofitted to an existing building.

1.11 RAMPS

Many ramps are intended to provide access to facilities for persons with disabilities, particularly those in wheelchairs. As such, specific requirements must be followed regarding dimensions, slope, and handrails for these components.

Ramp slopes are calculated by rise (vertical distance) over run (the length of the ramp) (Figure 1.37).

The slope should be no greater than 1 (vertical) × 8 (horizontal), or 7.1°. Ramps used for individuals with disabilities should have a slope no greater than 1 × 12 (4.8°), with slopes between 1:16 (3.6°) and 1:20 (2.9°) being optimal (NFPA, 2000; ADA, 1991). Figure 1.38 and Table 1.1 describe ramp slope and ramp slope conversions, respectively.

1.11.1 Ramp Design

The following additional guidelines apply:

- In general, a clear width of at least 36 in. should be present (ANSI A117.1), and no projections should extend into that space. This provides

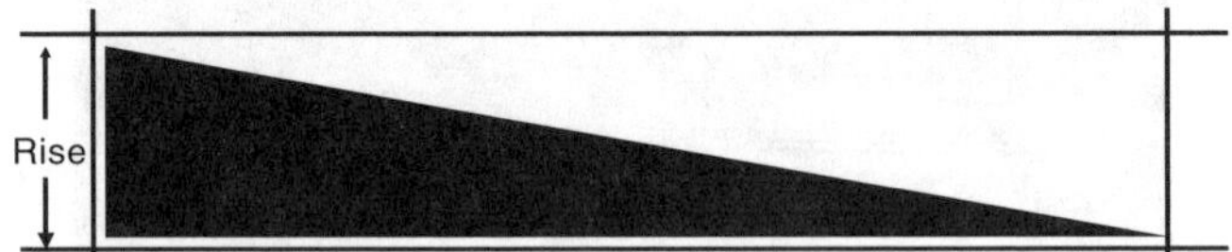

FIGURE 1.38 Slope is rise (height) over run (distance).

TABLE 1.1
Ramp Slope Conversions

Slope Ratio	Degrees	Notes
1:4	14	
1:6	9.5	
1:8	7.1	Maximum pedestrian ramp slope
1:10	5.7	
1:12	4.8	Maximum handicap new construction
1:15	3.8	
1:20	2.9	Walkway

sufficient width to permit the passage of a wheelchair. NFPA 101 requires new ramps and Class A ramps to be 44 in. minimum clear width, but permit Class B ramps to be as narrow as 30 in. Clear width and other ramp dimensions can also vary according to NFPA 101, depending on the occupancy.

- For 180° turns, ramp width must be at least 42 in. and at least 48 in. at the turn per ANSI A117.1 (see Figure 1.40).
- Unless a landing is present, the ramp must be a continuous, uniform slope.
- Handrails should be provided for ramps with a rise over 6 in.

Figure 1.39 illustrates a poorly designed ramp.

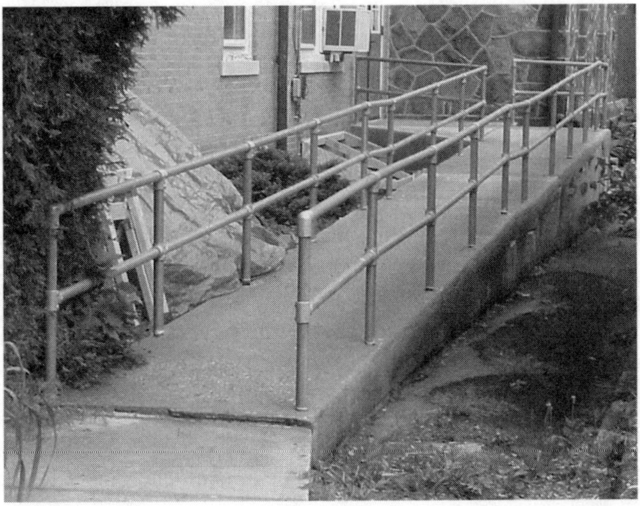

FIGURE 1.39 A poorly designed ramp. For starters, the slope is uneven and a tripping hazard is present at the base of the ramp.

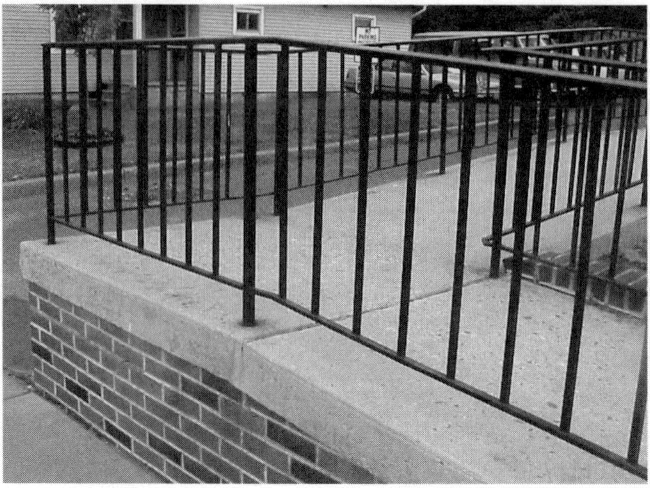

FIGURE 1.40 A good example of a ramp with a single turn.

1.11.2 Ramp Landings

- Ramp landings must be present at the top and bottom, and at doors opening onto the ramp.
- The landing slope should be no steeper than 1:48 and should be at least the same width as the ramp. The landing should be at least 60 in. long (in the direction of travel). For NPFA 101, existing ramp landings need not meet this requirement.

Figure 1.40 is an example of a ramp with a single turn.

1.12 FLOOR MATS/ENTRANCES AND EXITS

Entrance and exit areas are critical in controlling slip, trips, and falls because the concentrations of traffic and surface transitions are usually high. The exposure is highest in these areas because they constitute bottlenecks. Congestion is greater, contributing to the potential for pushing and tripping. Also, a high degree of surface wear occurs (which makes the walkway surfaces smoother and less tractive), as well as a higher concentration of water, dirt, and other contaminants from the footwear of people traversing that small area.

1.12.1 General Precautions

To reduce the potential for falls in these areas, consider the following:

- Identify surfaces with excessive smoothness and other defects. Changes in surface transitions can be of more concern than changes in levels.

This affects the "expectation" of the individual and often leads to stumbles and falls.

- Ensure door closure mechanisms are not forceful enough to knock someone over.
- Saddle (doorsill) height is a factor. To minimize an unexpected condition, it should be flush with the floor. The maximum safe height is $^3/_4$ in. (1.9 cm). Saddles should slope at the edges to avoid tripping hazards, and should be grooved or otherwise made slip resistant. Saddles should be secured tightly to the floor.
- Consider the impact of transitions between different types of floor surfaces, particularly transitions to extremes (e.g., very low to very high traction, or the reverse), which may present the pedestrian with an unexpected condition, thus increasing the likelihood of a fall.

1.12.2 Minimizing Contaminants

Entrances and exits should be designed to minimize slip and fall potential due to tracking in ice and snow on each visitor's footwear. Ideally, a grate system with a catch basin should be used in high-traffic situations to allow moisture removal from footwear. The grates should be placed perpendicular to the direction of travel. If this is not possible, mats should be used. The importance of proper mat selection and maintenance cannot be overstated. Mats of inappropriate design or poorly maintained mats can increase the hazard instead of mitigating it. Unless floor mats are engineered to wear and are properly cleaned on a consistent schedule, their ability to control the entry of contaminants will be significantly diminished because:

- Dust, dirt, and other contaminants in buildings are tracked into buildings from the outside 70 to 80% of the time.
- One square yard of commercial carpet can accumulate 1 1b of dirt a week and up to 2 lbs a week in wet weather.
- Only 10% of dirt is removed from floor mats with a vacuum cleaner.

Properly cleaned floor mats can catch approximately 70% of the dust tracked into a facility. Floor mats protect high-traffic areas and carpets from wear and tear. Because they absorb water, mud, and internally generated soil, floor mats also minimize conditions that can contribute to slips and falls. Floor mats can be used effectively in many areas, including front and rear entrance and exit doors, checkout counter areas, restrooms, kitchens, and around vending machines and water fountains.

1.12.3 Mat Design

Floor mats that are designed for removal of dust, dirt, and moisture from the shoe bottom are distinct from other types of floor coverings. Scatter rugs, carpet remnants, or cheap mats with borderless backing, vinyl backing, or no backing do not efficiently

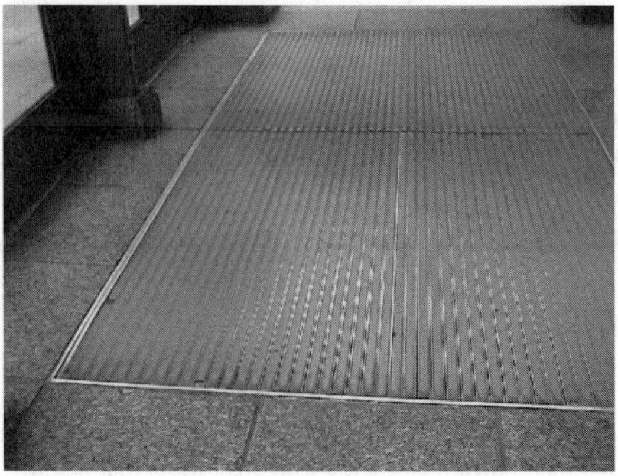

FIGURE 1.41 Good design for initial entrance matting: recessed, porous, and in good repair.

remove contaminants that accumulate on footwear bottoms, nor are they designed to minimize tripping or sliding underfoot.

The edging should be beveled in order to provide a smooth transition from the floor to the mat. Mats should be replaced before they become dog-eared. In most cases, the best solution is to use heavy-duty entrance mats that are constructed with a type of wire mesh that allows moisture and contaminants to drop away from the footwear (Figure 1.41).

1.12.4 Mat Design and Arrangement

One of the most effective arrangements is to have an embedded coarse mat in the entry/foyer area and a long runner mat (beveled and less coarse) as a runoff mat from the entryway into the building. This approach allows the bulk of contaminants to be removed by the abrasive mat, with the absorptive mat removing any residue. In cold weather, this order should be reversed. Figure 1.42 depicts such an arrangement.

Some mats are designed with nubbins, which are small rubber protrusions on the underside. These are intended to provide a degree of traction in order to avoid mat slippage when walked upon. Such designs are not appropriate on hard, smooth surfaces because the nubbins can compress from pressure and create ripples in the mat. This is especially the case when heavy objects, such as carts, are rolled across the mat.

Avoid stacking mats in use. This option might be considered when a mat has become saturated and, instead of removing and replacing it, another is placed on top. This increases the potential for tripping due to the substantially higher or uneven edge against the floor, however, and is more prone to rippling.

Mats are more likely to slide when dust and dirt accumulates under the mat due to inadequate cleaning of the floor underneath. Smooth-backed mats are the most susceptible to sliding under these conditions. The primary solutions are to ensure that mats are of the appropriate design for the flooring, and that cleaning is sufficient to preclude an accumulation of dust and dirt under the mat.

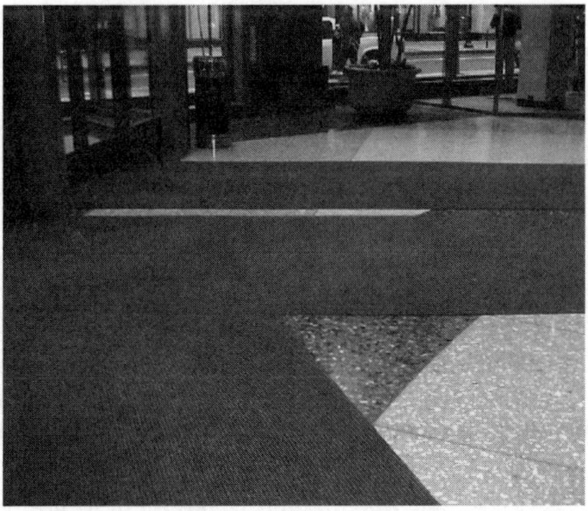

FIGURE 1.42 Good arrangement for second-tier matting that is strategically placed to cover natural pedestrian paths.

1.12.5 Mat Storage

Mat curling presents a tripping hazard. To reduce the potential for mat curling, mats should be rolled properly. The optimal method is to alternate rolling: each time the mat is rolled, alternate between front out and back out.

1.12.6 Mat Size

The Carpet and Rug Institute (CRI) *Commercial Carpet Maintenanc*e *Manual generally* defines an entrance (or soil wipe-off) area as the 90 ft^2 (6 ft × 15 ft) at building exterior entrances, where most tracked-in soil is deposited. CRI research shows that 80% of the soil brought into any building is trapped within the first 15 ft on a carpeted surface. A 10-ft^2 soil track-off region can also be found where the carpet and hard surfaces meet at main internal doorways, and a 40-ft^2 area in 6-ft wide main corridors.

Many commercial and institutional property owners and managers buy mats that are too small to be effective. CRI recommends selecting mats long enough to take two full steps (6 to 8 ft) before stepping onto other floor surfaces.

1.12.7 Protection of Hard Flooring Surfaces

Hard-surface floor coverings trap little dirt and moisture, allowing dirt, oily soil, and moisture to spread. The Resilient Floor Covering Institute (RFCI) states that accumulated soil diminishes the appearance of resilient flooring. RFCI's maintenance guide reports, "Preventing abrasive dirt from being tracked onto the surface of flooring is critical to prolong the life of resilient flooring. The use of walk-off mats at entrances is an effective way to prevent scratches and stains caused by tracked-in material from outside."

CRI's *Floor Covering Maintenance for School Facilities* states that daily maintenance of hard-surface floor covering presents a greater challenge than carpeted surfaces. Hard-surface flooring must receive constant care because of its inability to hide soil; the finish is also easily damaged by dry, gritty particulate soil and dirt. Recommended daily maintenance includes dry and wet mopping as well as spot mopping. Some high-traffic areas might require dust mopping several times a day. Strategically placed floor mats, which remove dirt and moisture deposits from footwear bottoms, reduce the need for more clean-up labor.

1.12.8 Mat Cleaning Guidelines

To maintain designed slip resistance, mats should receive scheduled cleanings of appropriate frequency based on the conditions to which they are subject. CRI's manual for school facilities states, "Walk-off mats should be cleaned frequently. Once a walk-off mat becomes filled with soil, the soil will then transfer to the soles of shoes and spread throughout the facility."

Entrance Mats — Take mats outside and shake them to remove excess dirt and debris. If necessary, use a hose (avoid extremely high pressure or high temperatures) to wash them off. Allow carpeted mats to dry before bringing them back inside.

Carpet Mats — Carpet mats can be cleaned the same way as carpeting. Vacuum them daily, and extract or shampoo them when dirt builds up.

Molded Rubber and PVC Anti-Fatigue Mats (designed for wet areas) — Use a high-pressure hose (not to exceed 1800 psi) and hot water (max 160°F) to remove oils. For best results, use a mild soap or detergent with a pH between 4.0 and 9.0 to clean the mats. Do not use steam, degreasers, or caustic chemicals. Do not machine wash or mechanically scrub the mats.

— Sweep regularly or dry mop the surface. These mats can be wet mopped with mild soap or detergent. For best results, use a detergent with a pH between 4.0 and 9.0.

Runner Mats — Sweep the surface with a broom or vacuum. Some runners can also be wet mopped with mild soap.

Electro-Static Discharge (ESD) Mats — ESD mats are designed to control the generation of static electricity. It is important to regularly sweep or dry mop the surface of ESD mats. Also, wet mop or wipe off with mild soap or a static control cleaning solution that will not leave a residue, so the mat will continue to work well.

For more information about floor mat design, maintenance, and professional mat services, visit the Textile Rental Services Association (TRSA) at http://www.trsa.org.

1.13 BATHROOMS

For durability, appearance, and ease of cleaning, glazed ceramic or similar tile is the flooring of choice in bathrooms. Untreated, this type of flooring commonly exhibits low slip resistance in wet conditions — a frequent occurrence. In some cases, mats are placed at sinks where water is most likely to reach the floor; however, rarely are the facilities to dry hands adjacent to the sink area. Paper towel dispensers and blowers are usually near the entrance or elsewhere, requiring travel with wet hands to that location, trailing water along the way. A simple change in arrangement can significantly reduce the exposure to falls.

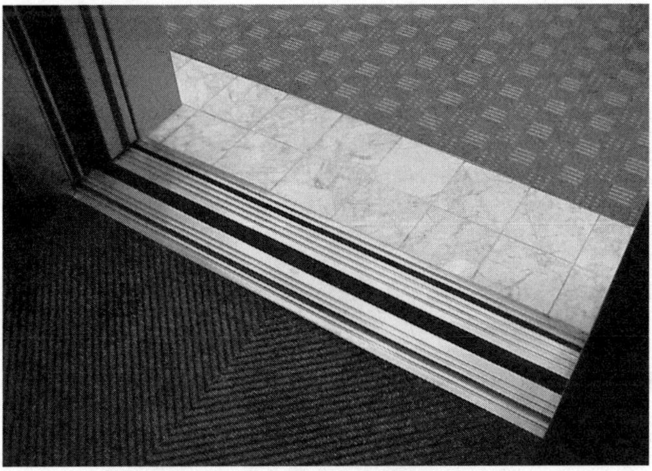

FIGURE 1.43 Fairly wide space between the elevator car and the floor. Multiple floor types can increase the potential for falls.

The bottom of bathtubs and showers are frequent sites of falls. These areas should not be smooth. Instead, they should be textured with appliques, treatments, or embedded patterns.

1.14 ELEVATORS

- Elevators need to be adjusted to be even and level with the floor surface.
- Space between the elevator car and the floor should be minimal (see Figure 1.43).
- Changes in floor surfaces in the elevator/lobby area should be minimal and, if present, clearly marked or differentiated.

1.15 ESCALATORS

- Warning signs should be provided to discourage or prohibit the use of strollers, caution about high-heeled shoes, and advise users to hold onto the handrail (see Figure 1.45).
- There should be emergency shutdown procedures in place.
- Where no other physical barrier is present, child guards should be provided at the entrance points of each escalator. These are designed to prevent children from holding onto and attempting to ride up on the outside of the escalator and becoming injured (see Figure 1.44 and Figure 1.46).
- ANSI A117.1 specifies that escalator handrails should be between 33 in. and 42 in.

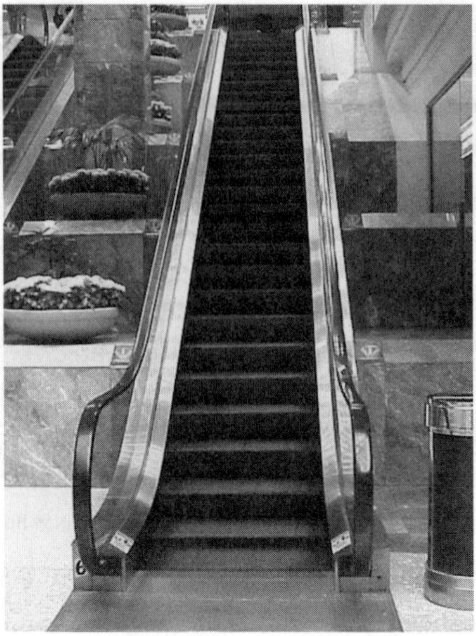

FIGURE 1.44 Well-arranged escalator. Barriers behind act as child guards.

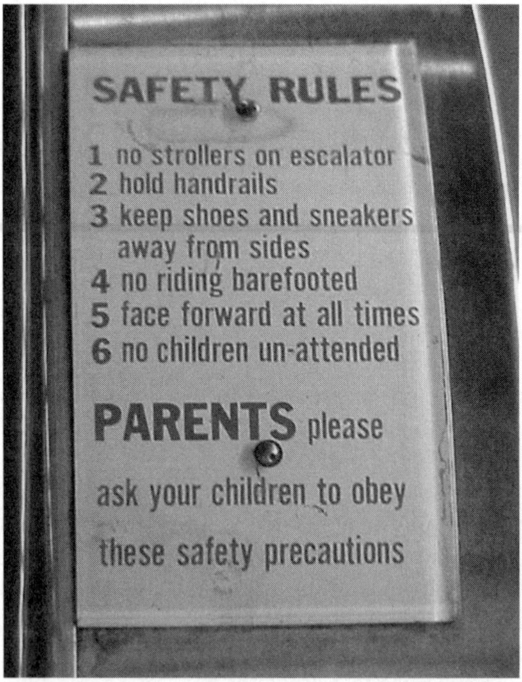
SAFETY RULES
1 no strollers on escalator
2 hold handrails
3 keep shoes and sneakers away from sides
4 no riding barefooted
5 face forward at all times
6 no children un-attended
PARENTS please
ask your children to obey
these safety precautions

FIGURE 1.45 Well-presented posted safety warnings.

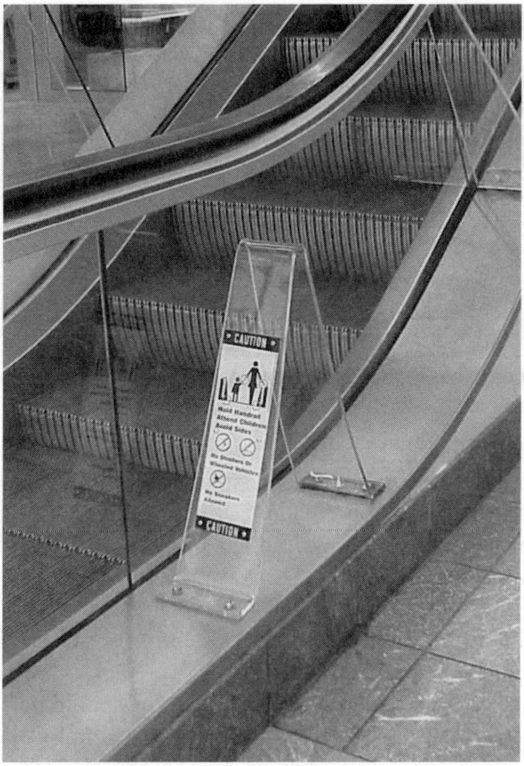

FIGURE 1.46 A standard child guard arrangement.

1.16 CARPET

In terms of slip resistance, carpet is one of the best walking surfaces that can be employed. Carpets have the added benefit of eliminating the problem of reflected glare associated with hard surface floors, which reduces visual disorientation and subsequent falls (see Figure 1.47 and Figure 1.48).

Some precautions should be kept in mind when using carpet:

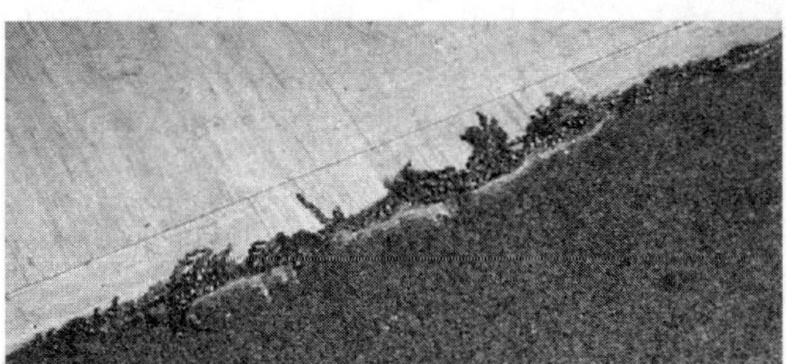

FIGURE 1.47 Carpet in poor stages of repair.

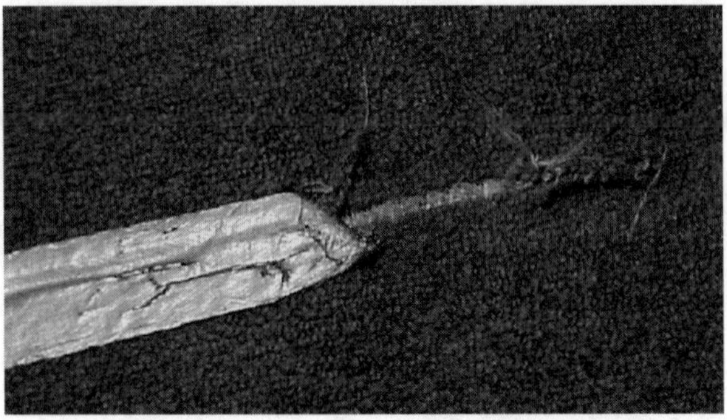

FIGURE 1.48 Carpet in poor stages of repair.

- Carpets should be checked for wear and looseness and repaired as necessary. Optimally, such conditions should not be permitted to develop.
- Just as with any other type of floor covering, carpets need to kept clean and free of debris, including granular material (e.g., sand, dirt) and wet contamination (e.g., water, oil).
- It is believed that the use of red carpet on steps (especially under low lighting conditions) inhibits depth perception, resulting in a disproportionately high potential for falls.
- Avoid "busy" carpet patterns. Instead, patterns should be subtle with low-contrast colors. High-contrast patterns tend to diminish an individual's ability to judge perspective, such as stair heights and other changes in the level of walking surfaces.

1.17 ACCESSIBILITY

Special access for individuals with disabilities should be evaluated for slip, trip, and fall hazards. Instead of just performing ADA compliance assessments, the focus should be to identify the potential for loss due to the inability of the facility to provide for adequate safe access of the disabled. For instance, the lack of entrance ramps and passenger loading areas may result in a person using a wheelchair to attempt to go over curbing to get to a sidewalk or entrance; this may result in a fall. Lack of room accommodations in a hotel, such as showers equipped for the handicapped, may force use of a conventional shower, which may contribute to a fall for a handicapped person.

Extensive design specifications are available on accessibility from references on the ADA (http://www.usdoj.gov/crt/ada/adahom1.htm) and ANSI A117.1 (http://www.ansi.org) (see Figure 1.49).

1.18 SIGNAGE

Signage should be provided where appropriate, considering changes in the type of floor surface, levels, trip hazards, and other conditions that the pedestrian would not expect to encounter.

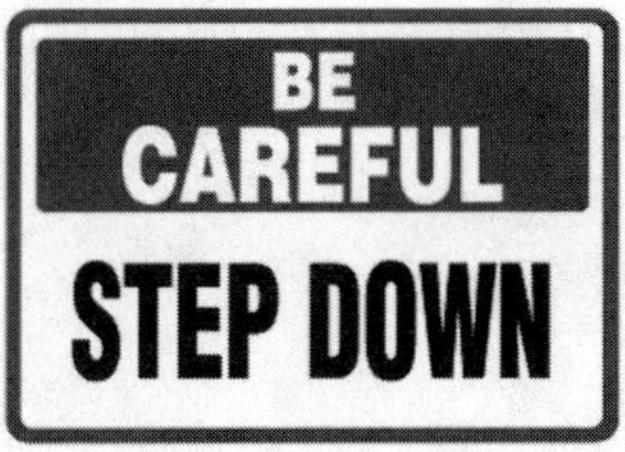

FIGURE 1.49 A typical design for signage to notify pedestrians of an unexpected change in walkway conditions.

Unfortunately, property owners often go to great expense to provide signs that blend into the environment. This negates the effectiveness of signs because they must be visible in order to be observed.

In selecting effective signage, signs must be understandable, legible, visible, and in compliance with legal standards. Consider the likelihood of multilingual and illiterate individuals. In these instances pictorial or multilingual signs may be most appropriate.

The Occupational Safety and Health Administration (OSHA) (29 CFR 1910.144) provides guidance on the proper design for safety signage:

- *Danger Signs* indicate immediate dangers and whether special precautions are necessary. Colors should be red, black, and white.
- *Caution Signs* warn against potential hazards or caution against unsafe practices. Colors should be yellow (background) and black with yellow letters (panel). Letters used against the yellow background must be black.
- *Safety Instruction Signs* should be used where a need exists for general instructions related to safety. Colors should be white (background) and green with white letters (panel). Letters against the white background must be black.

OSHA 29 CFR 1910.145 states that yellow shall be used for designating caution and for marking hazards, including stumbling, falling, and tripping.

Special consideration should also be given to those areas where guests need special warnings. For example, these areas might include prohibiting the use of strollers and the wearing of high heels. Other examples include signs reminding building occupants to use handrails, warning of icy conditions or a slippery ramp, pointing to a step up or a step down, and general guidance in congested or otherwise more hazardous areas to watch one's step. Signs of this type and many others are widely available (see Figure 1.50).

1.19 REFERENCE STANDARDS

1.19.1 NFPA International (formerly National Fire Protection Association)

For information about NFPA (http://www.nfpa.org), see Chapter 5.

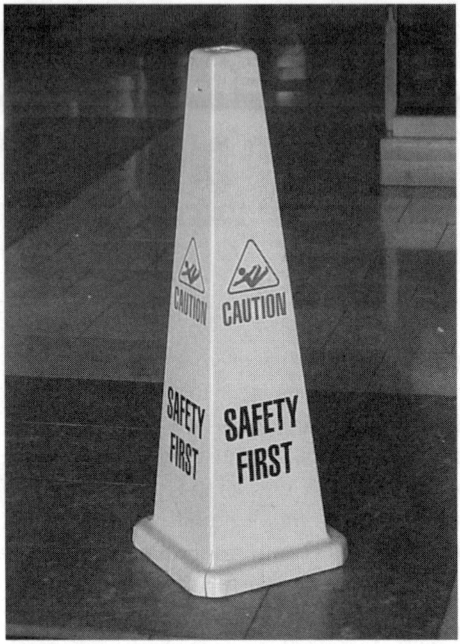

FIGURE 1.50 One of the many commonly used designs for warning cones to identify wet floor conditions.

1.19.1.1 NFPA 101 Life Safety Code (2000)

Although it is designed for building fire safety, this code also includes many well-founded principles of stair, ramp, and other walkway surface component design. It is also a nationally recognized consensus standard that can carry much weight in the courtroom. It provides requirements based on the occupancy (e.g., health care, places of assembly, mercantile, residential) and whether the facility is new or existing construction.

NPFA 101 is updated every 3 years. Although the requirements of existing construction rarely change, those for new construction may change significantly.

1.19.2 ASTM International (Formerly American Society of Testing and Materials)

For information about ASTM (http://www.astm.org), see Chapter 4.

1.19.2.1 ASTM F1637 Practice for Safe Walking Surfaces

This is a brief but useful document providing good design guidelines for all types of walkway surface components. It is updated periodically by ASTM under the jurisdiction of Technical Committee F13 Pedestrian/Walkway Safety and Footwear.

1.19.3 American National Standards Institute (ANSI)

For information about ANS I(http://www.ansi.org), see Chapter 5.

1.19.3.1 ICC/A117.1

The International Code Council (see Section 1.19.5) acts as secretariat for this standard, known as ADA-ANSI A117.1-1980, Accessible and Usable Buildings and Facilities. It provides specifications on making facilities accessible by persons with disabilities. There are two versions of the same standard with clear design guidelines for such components as ramps, landings, and curb cutouts. The ANSI 1996 edition is the most current, but the ADA edition is the most enforceable.

1.19.4 Occupational Safety and Health Administration (OSHA)

For more information about OSHA, go to http://www.osha.gov.

1.19.4.1 1910, Subpart D — Workplace Walking and Working Surfaces

Subpart D provides dimensional criteria for walkway components, including ramps, stairs, railings, and ladders.

1.19.5 Model Building Codes (IBC, BOCA, NBC, SBC, UBC)

The primary building code organizations in the U.S. are:

- Building Officials and Code Administrators, which promulgates the BOCA or National Building Code (NBC) (http://www.bocai.org/)
- Southern Building Code Congress International, which promulgates the Southern Building Code (SBC) (http://www.sbcci.org/)
- International Conference of Building Officials, which promulgates the Uniform Building Code (UBC) (http://www.icbo.org/)
- International Code Council, which promulgates the International Building Code (IBC) — The IBC was developed in a joint effort of the three primary U.S. building code organizations. Established in 1994 as a nonprofit organization, the objective of the ICC is to develop a single set of comprehensive and coordinated national model construction codes (http://www.intlcode.org/).
- National Fire Protection Association (NFPA 5000) (http://www.nfpa.org/)

Primary specifications relating to slip resistance and dimensional criteria for pedestrian safety are contained in Section 10 — Means of Egress. In general, the dimensional guidelines for ramps, stairs, handrails, guards, and other building features related to pedestrian safety are consistent among the various building codes, and with the NFPA Life Safety Code — Means of Egress.

Unlike NFPA 101, the model building codes address only new construction; however, states and even municipalities adopt different codes and different versions as well. The specific version of the model building code may have modifications in your local area. See Exhibit 1.2 for a summary of state-mandated building codes. These are perhaps the most important standards from a litigation standpoint, so it is essential that each facility complies with the appropriate building code.

1.19.6 ASME International (formerly American Society of Mechanical Engineers)

Founded in 1880, ASME (http://www.asme.org) is a nonprofit educational and technical organization servicing a worldwide membership of 125,000. It promulgates and maintains numerous standards involving the design, inspection, maintenance, and testing of escalators, elevators, and moving walks.

EXHIBIT 1.1
SLIP AND FALL SELF-ASSESSMENT CHECKLIST

SLIP AND FALL SELF-ASSESSMENT CHECKLIST

Facility Name:	Completed By:	Date:

INTERIOR

		Good	Fair	Poor	N/A
1.	**Facility Design & Arrangement**				
	- Stairs (non-slip, well-maintained, uniform tread & riser)				
	- Handrails (between 34-42" high, graspable, always within reach, sturdy)				
	- Elevators (level, minimal n floor surfaces minimal/marked)				
	- Entrances/Exits (non-slip, level, inclement weather measures)				
	- Entrance Mats (recessed, appropriate size, no "dog-eared" edges				
	- Lighting Adequate & Maintained				
	- Floor Levels/Surface Transitions (marked, unobstructed)				
2.	**Spill Program/Housekeeping**				
	- Response Time Standard Reasonable				
	- Appropriate Barriers/Signage Used				
	- Department Responsible Appropriate (Security &/or Housekeeping)				
	- Interim Measures Prior to Spill Clean-Up In Effect				
3.	**Incident Reporting/Investigation**				
	- Response Time Standard (specify):				
	- Department Responsible Appropriate/Trained in 1st Aid & CPR (Security)				
	- First Priority: Attend To Injured Person				
	- Obtain Facts About The Accident				
	- Obtain Witness Name, Address, Telephone Numbers				
	- Take Photograph Of Accident Scene				
	- Complete Written Report Of Findings				
	- Take Corrective Action To Prevent Re-occurrence				
4.	**Construction/Renovation/Special Event Planning**				
	- Department/Personnel Overseeing Activities (specify):				
	- Methods For Securing Areas From Public Access				
	- Adequacy Of Non-Public Areas (i.e. hazards to contractors on-site)				
5.	**Preventative/Other Programs**				
	- Plotting Facility Slip/Falls On Map				
	- Slip Meter Readings/Documentation (specify):				
	- Purchasing Controls In Place/Adequate (evaluate floor wax/finish)				
	- Subcontract Housekeeping/Maintenance (hold harmless/certificates of ins)				
	- Other Measures (specify):				

EXTERIOR

		Good	Fair	Poor	N/A
1.	**Design & Arrangement**				
	- Grading/Drainage (for ice/water accumulation)				
	- Sidewalks/Steps (level, non-slip, changes marked, handrails)				
	- Parking Lots (level, grading/drainage)				
	- Lighting Adequate/Footcandle Measurements Documented				
	- Shortcuts Minimized (landscaped to discourage access beyond sidewalks)				
2.	**Inspection/Maintenance**				
	- Self-Inspection/Corrective Action				
	- Maintenance Procedures (scheduled, prioritized action on work orders)				
	- Snow/Ice Removal Procedures				

SPACE FOR ADDITIONAL COMMENTS ON OTHER SIDE

Slip/Fall Self-Assessment Checklist
page two

Comments:

EXHIBIT 1.2
STATE-MANDATED BUILDING CODES[A]

State	State Code Name	Code Basis and Edition
Alabama	State of Alabama Building Code	SBC, 1994
Alaska	Uniform Building Code	UBC, 1997
Arizona	None	
Arkansas	Arkansas Fire Prevention Code	SBC, 1997
California	Title24	UBC, 1997
Colorado	CO Construction Code	UBC, 1997
Connecticut	State Building Code	NBC, 1990
Delaware	None	
Florida	SBC, EPCOT, SFBC	SBC, 1997
Georgia	GA Minimum Standards Code for Construction	SBC, 1997
Hawaii	None	
Idaho	None	
Illinois	None	
Indiana	Indiana Building Code	UBC, 1997
Iowa	None	
Kansas	None	
Kentucky	Kentucky Building Code	NBC, 1996
Louisiana	Standard Building Code	SBC, 1994
Maine	BOCA	NBC, 1993
Maryland	MD Building Performance Standards	NBC, 1996
Massachusetts	Massachusetts State Building Code	NBC, 1993
Michigan	Michigan Building Code	NBC, 1996
Minnesota	Minnesota State Building Code	UBC, 1997
Mississippi	None	
Missouri	None	
Montana	Administrative Rules of Montana	UBC, 1997
Nebraska	Uniform Building Code	UBC, 1997
Nevada	None	
New Hampshire	New Hampshire State Fire Code	NBC, 1996
New Jersey	NJ Uniform Construction Code	NBC, 1996
New Mexico	Uniform Building Code	UBC, 1997
New York	State Uniform Fire Prevention & Building Code	State, 1995
North Carolina	North Carolina State Building Code	SBC, 1994
North Dakota	North Dakota State Building Code	UBC, 1997
Ohio	Ohio Basic Building Code	NBC, 1996
Oklahoma	None	
Oregon	Oregon Specialty Codes	UBC, 1997
Pennsylvania	None	
Rhode Island	RI State Building Code	NBC, 1996
South Carolina	Standard Building Code	SBC, 1997
South Dakota	Uniform Building Code	UBC, 1994
Tennessee	Standard Building Code	SBC, 1997
Texas	None	
Utah	Uniform Building Code	UBC, 1997
Vermont	Vermont Fire Prevention & Building Code	NBC, 1987
Virginia	Virginia Uniform Statewide Building Code	NBC, 1996
Washington	Uniform Building Code	UBC, 1997
West Virginia	State Building Code	NBC, 1996
Wisconsin	Wisconsin Building Code	State
Wyoming	Uniform Building Code	UBC, 1997
District of Columbia	BOCA 1990	NBC, 1990

*excerpted and edited from the Institute for Business and Safety Summary of State-Mandated Building Codes (http://ww.ibhs.org)

2 Management Controls

2.1 INTRODUCTION

A well-designed facility can still be subject to frequent fall accidents if appropriate management controls are not in place. The purpose of management controls is to maintain the facility in a condition as free from hazards as reasonably possible. The extent of management controls considered adequate depends on a variety of factors, including: the size of the facility; the amount of foot traffic; the familiarity of building occupants with their surroundings; the type of hazards; and the scope of programs implemented by other similar facilities. Thus, programs considered adequate for a small manufacturing facility would be vastly different from what might be suitable for a large hotel. The manufacturing facility would have low foot traffic, mostly from employees familiar with the facility, while the hotel would likely have very high foot traffic, mostly from visitors who are unfamiliar with their surroundings.

2.2 ENGINEERING PRECEPT

When designing your facility and developing your management control programs, it is helpful to remember this engineering precept: "design to the lowest common denominator."

Assume that anyone, in any condition, could enter your facility. Once someone enters the facility and becomes a building occupant, management assumes some degree of responsibility for the safety of the surroundings. Consider that someone who is disabled or impaired, including someone who is moderately ambulatory or nonambulatory, blind, or deaf, may be present. Consider that someone under the influence of alcohol or drugs — prescription, over-the-counter, or illegal — may be present. Consider that someone (probably many people) who is distracted or stressed with other things on his or her mind may be present.

Any of these categories present an increased risk of injury, particularly falls. As such, an effective development method is to use these scenarios to design, implement, and test your management programs.

2.3 BEHAVIORAL SAFETY AND PEDESTRIAN TRAFFIC FLOW

High traffic flow areas are especially susceptible to trips/falls. These areas should be observed closely, and traffic flows should be determined for various times of the day. Management procedures should then be evaluated to ensure that adequate controls are in place to address the various issues that may arise.

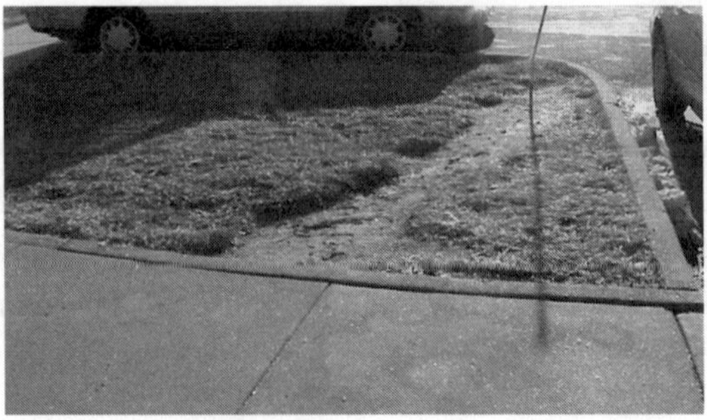

FIGURE 2.1 Actual pedestrian traffic flow is clearly indicated by this well-worn shortcut from parking lot to the sidewalk.

Analyze losses according to time of day, day of the week, or similar criteria to determine if congestion related to traffic flow is a factor in slip/fall incidents. Analyze measures taken to control large crowds.

Consider putting controls in place to guide large crowds safely through the walking area. Use fencing for outside conditions or other forms of guide rails both inside and outside; however, barriers and visual cues, such as lighting and signage in place, may not produce the desired behavior. In general, it is human nature to take the shortest and easiest path to a destination.

2.3.1 Natural Paths/Observation

After identifying the time periods representing the highest exposure (based on volume and/or incidents), spend some time watching how people move; for instance, look for worn paths cutting across open areas where the sidewalk turns (see Figure 2.1).

Observe high traffic flow areas closely. Traffic flows should be determined for various times of the day.

Management procedures should then be evaluated to ensure that adequate controls are in place to address the various issues that may arise.

Consider the following:

- Wear and tear on floor surfaces creating depressions and worn carpet surfaces
- Controls in place to guide large crowds safely through the walking area
- Use of fences for outside conditions or other forms of guide rails in place both inside and outside

2.3.2 Adapt or Adopt

Where practical, it is best to adopt the path created by human behavior. Thus, as presented in Figure 2.2, consider paving that worn path and making it suitable for pedestrian use.

Sidewalks and other pedestrian routes should be designed to use the most efficient path. This will reduce or eliminate the potential for pedestrians to shortcut

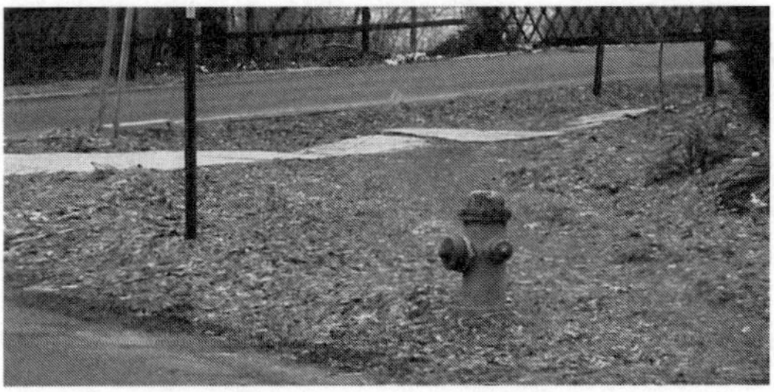

FIGURE 2.2 A more direct path, avoiding walking around the corner, is shown by this path.

into unintended and possibly dangerous areas. It is optimal to determine where and how people tend to walk and design these routes based on that behavior.

Once known, alternatives can be developed and again tested by observation.

2.4 INSPECTION AND MAINTENANCE PROGRAMS

A major cause of falls relates to pedestrians encountering unexpectedly slippery (usually wet) surfaces. Frequently, this is caused by insufficient maintenance of the building or equipment (e.g., leaks of pipes, hoses, tanks, roofs) or by belated detection of a condition (e.g., spills, overspray, entry of moisture at entrances). Thus, it could be argued that, in conjunction with proper facility design, superior maintenance and inspection programs are the most effective means of preventing conditions that result in slips and falls.

Management's inspection and maintenance programs must meet several criteria to be considered adequate. These programs must:

- Be of a scope commensurate to the size and occupancy of the facility — A large facility with vague, incomplete, or cursory programs will likely be unsuccessful in preventing or quickly correcting hazardous conditions.
- Be scheduled at a reasonable frequency — The longer that hazardous conditions are permitted to remain unabated, the greater the potential for an injury.
- Be consistently and uniformly applied — What you put in writing, you should follow through with. If, for example, your inspection program calls for three inspections a day of a given area, monitor to assure that three — not two — inspections are being performed.
- Involve not just the employees who are directly involved in administering the program, but all employees. The more eyes, the more quickly and thoroughly will substandard conditions be detected and corrected.
- Be well documented — Perhaps you have inspected three times a day, but you should also have documentation that you did.

2.5 SELF-INSPECTION PROGRAMS

For most facilities, there should be a formal program in place to inspect for slip-and-fall-related exposures. This control may be included in a facility inspection or review that covers slip and fall hazards as well as other issues (e.g., security, housekeeping, life safety). Consistently documented inspections can help establish the presence or absence of those hazards.

To establish a reasonable schedule for self-inspection, one option is to plot each slip and fall incident on a map of the facility. This may provide clear indications of areas that need attention.

Other ways of establishing reasonable self-inspections schedules include:

- Adopting industry-specific standards developed and promoted by industry associations
- Consulting with other similar facilities nearby to determine their frequency and scope of self-inspection

These two options can be particularly beneficial because, in the event of a lawsuit, the plaintiff's counsel may compare the quality of your program with that of your industry and other facilities like yours.

2.6 SPILL AND WET PROGRAM

Slips on wet surfaces are a leading cause of severe injuries. For operations that have this substantial exposure, policies and procedures should be in place to deal with spills, wet surfaces from inclement weather, and any other source of water or other wet walkway surfaces.

A spill and wet program is essentially a customized, focused, housekeeping program designed to provide prompt detection, response, and corrective action.

Sufficient equipment and materials should be available to handle any wet problem that is likely to be encountered. Signs and barriers should be employed. For spills, there should be interim measures in effect to temporarily protect the area until cleanup is complete. This will usually consist of yellow cones, triangles, or other placards. These barriers should mark off the area boundaries in order to notify pedestrians, coming from any direction, of the hazard. Barriers should not be removed until the area is not only clean, but is also completely dry (see Figure 2.3).

For facilities with a frequency of spill and wet exposures, standards for response time and cleanup should be established, measured, and documented. Once put in writing, it is essential that those procedures be observed.

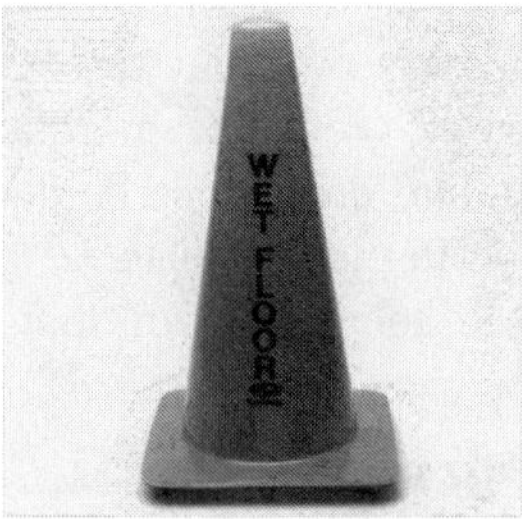

FIGURE 2.3 A basic component of an effective spill and wet program is to preclude pedestrian access by fully sectioning off wet floor areas by using readily identifiable barriers such as wet floor signs/cones.

2.7 RECOMMENDED PRACTICES FOR SNOW REMOVAL

Ice and snow management should be considered emergency work, and the property should be cleared day or night. Removal of snow from walkways and parking lots is essential to the safety of employees and visitors. Snow removal efforts should be performed as expeditiously as conditions and resources allow.

The planning and preparation process is made difficult by the varied conditions that can be presented during each storm. Variables in moisture content, temperature, wind, depth of snow, and rate of snowfall affect removal efforts. For example, if there is ice buildup under the snow, it may be prudent to leave the snow on the ice until warmer weather arrives. If the wind is blowing strongly, the removal effort is a judgment call. Light snow can be removed in greater depths with a broom than wet, heavy snow.

The use of ice-melt chemicals, has in some cases, replaced the traditional salt or sand. Although some of these chemicals are effective and appropriate, others can create an unexpected slipping hazard. Anhydrous chemicals are hydrophilic and should be avoided. Under certain conditions, as the ice is melted, these chemicals can combine with the water to become a slippery surface.

2.7.1 Objectives

Realizing that the expectation of employees and visitors may be broom-clean and dry pavement 24 hours a day, 365 days a year, we try to do what we reasonably can. When grounds maintenance receives a concern, it should be investigated and efforts made to improve the situation in a reasonable time. Primary objectives of snow and ice removal are:

- Safety for motorists and pedestrians
- Safety for the grounds maintenance personnel who are performing the work
- Protection of landscaping and property

2.7.2 Personnel and Responsibilities

2.7.2.1 Facility Manager

The facility manager should make decisions about snow removal efforts after careful consideration of all variables. The facilities manager (or designee) may declare an ice/snow removal emergency. This may require the closure of parking facilities and the removal of parked vehicles that interfere with ice and snow removal operations.

2.7.2.2 Custodians

Custodians in each building should be responsible for removal of snow at the building entrances for a distance of about 6 feet from the buildings. The custodial staff should also be responsible for removal of snow from steps at the main entrances to buildings. Steps should be kept as ice-free as possible.

2.7.2.3 Grounds Maintenance Staff

This staff should be responsible for deicing and snow removal of primary and secondary sidewalks, Americans with Disabilities Act (ADA) ramps and curb cuts, weather-exposed stairwells, and parking lots. The grounds maintenance staff should assure that, once the melt has started, curb inlets, catch basins, and trench drains will be unobstructed to further the melt runoff.

2.7.2.4 Contracted Snow Removal

Caution should be exercised when contracting snow removal. Inquiries should be made regarding the workload of the contractor. Obtain reasonable assurance that the contractor has not secured so many jobs that it is unable to fulfill its responsibilities in a timely manner, or to the specifications of the contract.

If engaged, snow removal contractors should be responsible by contract to remove snow from parking lots, parking lot entrances, and loading docks. The loading and hauling of snow may be required to clear adequate parking spaces.

2.7.3 Guidelines for Removal

The facilities manager should call for removal operations when there is more than 1 in. of snow accumulation, or sleet and iced-over conditions:

- Use brooms to clean sidewalks and walkways for snowfalls of less than 4 in.
- Use a skid steer loader on sidewalks and walkways if snowfall is 4 in. or greater.
- Sanding of roadways should be at the judgment of the grounds maintenance supervisor in consultation with the facilities manager and the police department.
- Snowfalls greater than 18 in. may require the assistance of a contractor to remove snow from parking lots. The facilities manager and grounds maintenance supervisor should make decisions about contracted snow removal.

After the snow stops falling, and after the major walks and roads are cleared, crews should concentrate on clearing snow from remaining areas and sanding as needed.

2.7.4 Priorities for Removal

1. Fire lanes must be open for emergency equipment. Fire hydrants must be free of snow and accessible at all times.
2. Main entrances, ADA ramps and curb cuts, weather-exposed stairs, and primary sidewalks and parking lots should be cleaned before the building opens.
3. Parking lots, secondary entrances, and other low-usage areas should be cleaned by noon.

For problem areas, close the area, or provide warning of the problem. For adverse situations, reasonable care and a special effort are expected.

When snow is removed during any time other than the normal working hours (e.g., weekend snow removal), the grounds maintenance supervisor should call all personnel to inform them of the best time to report to work. Contractors should remove snow from sidewalks on weekends on an as-needed basis. The grounds crew should be responsible for weekend snow removal if contractors are not engaged or not available.

2.7.5 Snow Storage

Generally, snow can be piled in the parking lots where removed:

- Snow should be piled at locations and in heights to avoid impairing visibility.
- Do not block storm drainage with snow piles.
- Do not pile snow on shrubs or ornamental trees.
- Do not block ADA curb cuts and parking spots with snow piles.
- Do not trap water around buildings with snow piles.
- Do not pile snow at a higher elevation or nearby pedestrian walkways, such that the melting snow would create runoff and present additional hazards upon freezing.

2.8 LIGHTING

A recent study (Davies et al., 2001) indicated that poor lighting significantly increased the risk of an underfoot accident. Gender was found to be an indicator, with women experiencing a substantially higher risk of such accidents than men. One of the researchers' conclusions was that wearing bifocal/varifocal eyeglasses increased the risk of "missed edge of" (step) accidents. Researchers suggested that two sets of eyewear (one for walking, another for reading and close work) might be effective in reducing this risk.

Most people lose visual acuity with age. By age 40, visual acuity is reduced by 10%, and is down 26% by age 60. Between ages 70 and 79, only 25% of people demonstrate normal 20/20 vision, and only 14% of those over age 80 have normal vision. This loss is more pronounced under low-light conditions. Color perception is also decreased as one grows older, as is depth perception. This condition lessens the ability to recognize and adapt to nonstandard stairs and ramps. Avoiding glare is particularly important for older individuals because the aging eye is less able to detect contrasts and does not adjust as rapidly to changes from light to dark. Focusing close-up and distinguishing contrasts is more difficult for older individuals, so more light is needed.

Poor lighting plays an increasing role in litigation for slip, trip, and fall accidents. Experts refer to the standards published by the Illuminating Engineering Society of North America (IESNA), which provides guidelines in footcandles for most occupancies and activities (http://www.iesna.org). The IESNA notes that the guidelines do not contemplate the age of occupants, acknowledging that the requirements of older individuals is markedly different for two reasons:

(1) There is a thickening of the yellow crystalline lens, which decreases the amount of light reaching the retina, increases scatter within the eye, and reduces the range of distances that can be properly focused, and (2) There is a reduction of pupil size, decreasing the amount of light reaching the retina.

2.8.1 Light Sources

Selecting the right type of light source is an important consideration. Studies show that the eye's response to color depends upon the amount of light available. The color sensitivity of the eye changes at different light levels. Under low light levels, the eye's sensitivity to yellow and red light is greatly reduced, while the response to blue light is greatly increased (see Figure 2.4).

2.8.1.1 Mercury Vapor

Mercury vapor lamps are known for their long life (24,000+ h) and good efficiency (31 to 63 LPW) as compared with incandescent lamps. Because of their long life, mercury vapor lamps are widely used in street lighting; approximately 75% of all street lighting is mercury vapor.

2.8.1.2 Metal Halide

Metal halide lamps are similar in design and operation to mercury vapor lamps. The efficiency of metal halide lamps (80 to 115 LPW) is approximately 50%

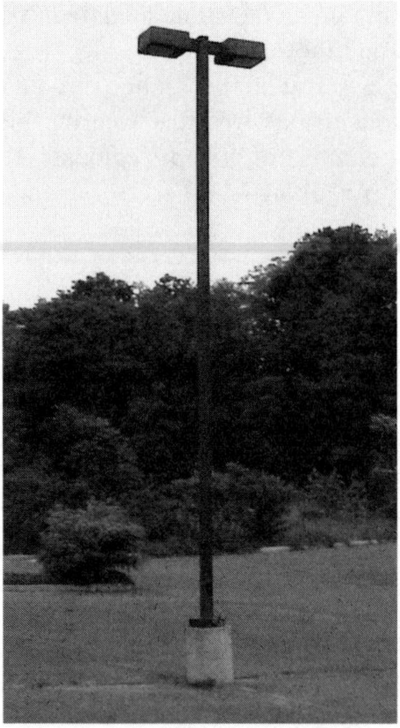

FIGURE 2.4 Lighting in parking lots should be over-designed to allow for time to change burned out bulbs and provide redundant light sources to avoid dependence on a single lighting unit..

higher than mercury vapor lamps, but metal halide has a much shorter lamp life (6000 h).

Metal halide lamps have strong light output in the blue, green, and yellow regions. The result is a high lumen output at all light levels. The blue light output of metal halide is in the high sensitivity region of the eye for low light levels. This means that the effective lumens actually increase for a metal halide lamp as the light level reduces and the eye shifts to a high blue or green sensitivity. Metal halide lamps are also less sensitive to temperature than, for example, fluorescents. Fluorescents are designed to perform optimally at around 70°F, and will show measurable decline in lumens in temperatures higher or lower than 70°F. Metal halide lamps, on the other hand, operate efficiently down to minus 40°F and are relatively unaffected by wide variations in ambient temperature.

2.8.1.3 High Pressure Sodium (HPS)

HPS lights have rapidly gained acceptance in the exterior lighting of parking areas, roadways and building exteriors because of their high efficiency. They operate on the same principles as mercury vapor and metal halide lamps. This type of lamp has a high efficiency (80 to 140 LPW), relatively good color rendition, long lamp life (24,000 h), and an excellent lumen depreciation factor that averages about 90% throughout its rated life.

Most of the output of sodium light sources is in the yellow region, giving very high lumen output under high light levels but poor output under low light levels. Consequently, high-pressure sodium lamps have high lumen ratings as perceived by the eye. On the other hand, under low light conditions, the effective lumens are greatly reduced because sodium produces little blue and green light.

2.8.2 Lighting Levels — Safety Only

The following are general guidelines on lighting levels, considered by the IESNA as the "absolute minimum for safety alone." Substantially higher levels of lighting are appropriate for many reasons, such as that needed for work activities and security. These bare minimum requirements will vary based upon the occupancy/activities, occupants, and site conditions.

Lighting is normally measured in terms of "footcandles" (fc), which is the amount of light given off by a candle at a distance of 1 ft. It can also be measured in "lux," (lx) in which 1 fc is equivalent to 10.76 lx (see Figure 2.5).

Interior lighting standards are relative to the hazard. The IESNA specifies the following "absolute minimums for safety alone": 2.0 fc for areas where there is a low level of activity, and 5.0 fc for areas where there is a high level of activity.

For *exterior lighting standards,* light meter readings must be done at night. In general, exterior areas of high pedestrian usage should be at least 0.9 fc, and 0.2 fc should be provided in areas of less use. Enclosed garages should be provided with at least 5 fc.

High intensity discharge (HID) lamps are recommended, which include mercury vapor, metal halide, and HPS.

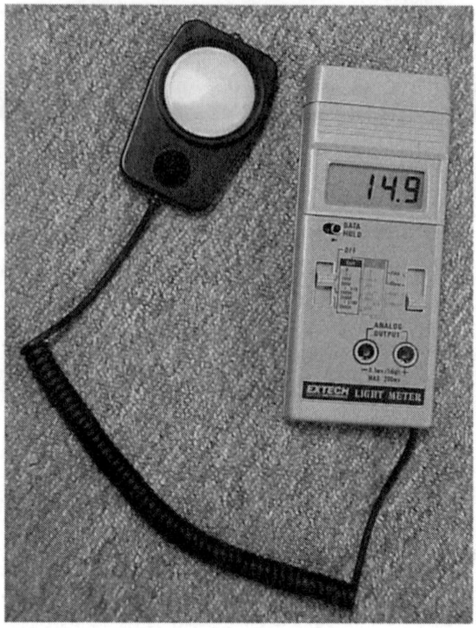

FIGURE 2.5 Digital light meters can provide light level readings in footcandle (fc) or lux (lx) scales.

2.8.3 Lighting Levels — Categories

In 1979, the IESNA developed recommended lighting levels based on a judgment of best practice for typical applications. Originally comprising nine categories, this tiered classification system was later revised to seven categories.

- Categories A, B, and C are for the purposes of "orientation and simple visual tasks," and specify the lowest levels of lighting.
- Categories D, E, and F are intended for "common visual tasks."
- Category G was created to address "visually demanding" tasks and specify the highest levels of illumination.

Categories A through C are of most interest with respect to fall prevention, as presented in Table 2.1. Examples of activities/areas within these categories are listed in Table 2.2.

TABLE 2.1
IESNA Lighting Categories A, B, and C

Category	Activity	Footcandles
For purposes of orientation and simple visual tasks		
A	Public spaces	3
B	Basic orientation for short visits	5
C	Working spaces for visual tasks	10

TABLE 2.2
IESNA Examples of Lighting Categories

Category	Activity and Occupancy
A	Dance Halls
	Hospital Corridors
	Houses of Worship Congregational Areas
	Museum Lobbies
	Toilets and Washrooms
B	Hospital Patient Rooms
	Library Bookstacks (Inactive)
	Merchandising Dressing Areas
	Service Space Stairways and Corridors
	Shopping Mall Main Concourse Areas
C	Educational Corridors
	Hotel Lobbies
	Merchandising General Display Areas
	Office Filing Areas
	Supermarkets

2.8.4 Lighting Transitions

Also of importance is the transitioning from a well-lit area to a low-light area, and vice versa. Even in people with excellent vision, it takes some time for the human eye to readjust to different lighting levels. Transitions between bright and dark areas should be as gradual as possible. Using various visual cues and barriers to slow pedestrian traffic flow can also assist by permitting more time for pedestrians to adjust to new light levels.

In addition to lighting levels and transitions, the adequacy of lighting conditions should include assessment and control of shadows and glare. Shadows can mask hazardous conditions, making them unexpected to the pedestrian. Glare, similar to transition extremes, can temporary impair the sight of pedestrians, increasing their potential for falling.

2.8.5 Maintenance

A well-designed lighting maintenance program is an important part of providing good visibility. Gradual accumulation of dust and dirt on fixture lenses and lamps reduces light output. Regularly scheduled cleaning and relamping, as well as prompt replacement of defective lenses and ballasts, can increase efficiency (see Figure 2.6). The lighting maintenance program should include the following elements:

- The extent and frequency of maintenance should be consistent with the manufacturer's specifications. Cleaning luminaires (casing and reflector) and replacing bulbs is essential to achieving the design efficiency and brightness.
- Where possible, weekly inspections of lighting should be performed, especially where maintenance logs show a trend of outages. An alternative

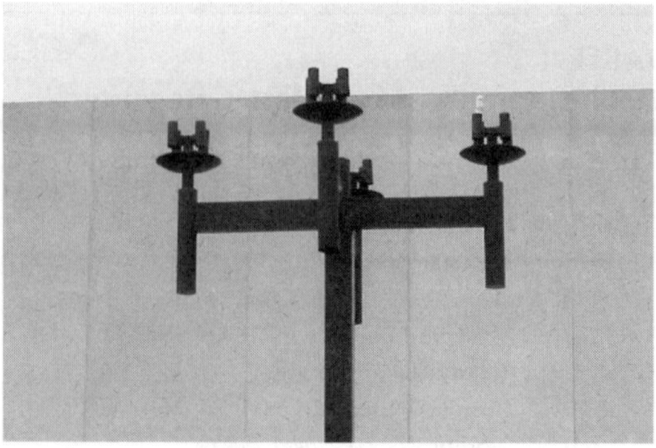

FIGURE 2.6 Of the 16 light sockets, only one has a bulb, significantly reducing lighting levels at night. Also, protective covers are not used.

is to provide monitoring by a computerized environmental control system that indicates when maintenance is required.

- It is also important that lighting is overdesigned for the area. The provision of supplemental or additional lights or bulbs will help ensure that sufficient lighting is available, even if one or two bulbs burn out or are vandalized.
- If timers instead of photoelectric sensors control lighting, procedures should be in place to adjust them consistent with seasonal time and light changes.

2.9 CONTRACTUAL RISK TRANSFER

An effective tool is risk transfer or risk sharing. Some facilities arrange to subcontract all or part of their floor housekeeping/care and snow removal activities. A "hold harmless" with language in your favor and adequate limits of liability is included, often with your company as an additional named insured to the contractor's policy. Claim activity should be monitored to ensure that claims for which the contractor is responsible are not being erroneously posted to your policy.

A limited risk transfer can be achieved by subcontracting normal maintenance with verification of liability insurance of adequate limits. When you are renovating properties or expanding operations, require adherence to specifications for slip resistance in purchasing contracts and require certification of the materials used.

Other risk transfer issues are related to slips, trips, and falls, including instances in which the tenant, instead of the property owner, is held liable for hazardous conditions in parking lots and on other walking surfaces. Responsibilities regarding maintenance, inspection, housekeeping, insurance, and related responsibilities should be clearly assigned in contractual agreements.

2.9.1 General Administrative Measures

Regardless of the size of the organization, a structured program for controlling contractual risk transfers is essential. All personnel who negotiate contracts should have those contracts reviewed by legal counsel. Exposures may be hidden in even the most "simple" of contracts.

Except when changes are made, boilerplate or "standard" contracts may need only auditing and monitoring after an initial in-depth review; however, other contracts are not "routine." It is critical to understand that risk transfer agreements are not always easily identified, are less easy to evaluate, and can be unexpectedly hazardous. Legal counsel should be responsible for reviewing and controlling such transfers, and must be given adequate opportunity to perform the difficult task of reviewing and interpreting each contract.

Even when you consider a contract to be simple, routine, or standard, you should always check with legal counsel to determine the best approach.

2.9.2 Specific Control Measures

A contract should always be reviewed prior to signing in order to provide an opportunity to submit recommendations to management on how to best handle the exposure posed by inappropriate provisions contained in the contract.

Reduce Exposures Assumed – Wherever possible, you may wish to narrow the scope of the transfer provision to what you know can be accommodated by your own insurance coverage. Be cautious about the number of contractual transfers simultaneously in effect because an excessive number may complicate business relationships and increase costs.

Judicious Retention of Exposures – Agreements may present exposures that the organization is willing to assume without calling upon another party's insurance. If retained, the exposures should be limited to those known to be low in expected frequency and severity, and free from potential catastrophe.

Insurance Transfer – To evaluate whether exposures will be covered by insurance, you must first be certain that coverage is available. The other party's applicable insurance coverage should also be examined and verified.

Dealing with "Unmanageable" Provisions – Even the best use of loss reduction, risk retention, and insurance may not be adequate to control some exposures transferred. Instead of rejecting the contract, management can seek to change or remove objectionable provisions. The success in making such changes, however, depends in large part on the bargaining strength of the parties and the importance of their contractual relationship to each of them.

Clarity of Contract Language – Contract language should always be written as clearly as possible; if the language is unclear, it must be revised.

2.9.3 Fundamental Guidelines

Make sure the indemnitor is financially able to stand behind its commitment. In considering recent court decisions, it is almost essential that the commitment be backed by adequate limits of insurance. Consult your licensed insurance professional for advice as to how much is adequate in any given situation.

Require a certificate of insurance for contractual liability coverage before contract operations begin. The certificate should clearly state that the issuer (or insurer) must provide at least 30 days automatic notice of cancellation, nonrenewal, or material change in coverage directly to you, the certificate holder. Merely obtaining a copy of the insurance policy will not provide notice of cancellation or coverage change. A system should be established to update all certificates prior to expiration, when a contract is renewed or open-ended, or when the contract exceeds the period covered by the certificate.

Where possible, be named as an additional insured and obtain a waiver of subrogation from insurers. Although being an additional insured may obligate the organization to pay premiums or require compliance with certain conditions following a loss, the advantages far outweigh the disadvantages. Unfortunately, this level of protection is not always available in the insurance marketplace.

2.10 CONSTRUCTION, RENOVATION, AND SPECIAL EVENT PLANNING

The potential for conditions creating slip and fall hazards should be considered in all construction and special event activities. This includes adequate staff to identify and correct such conditions, and controlled access to nonpublic and hazardous areas. Where practical, adequate physical barriers should be in place to secure hazardous areas from public access. Such activities usually call for increased inspection rounds and staffing.

Good guidance on appropriate controls for this type of exposure can be found in Occupational Safety and Health Administration (OSHA) 1926, Subpart M on Fall Protection. Although much of this section has to do with fall arrest systems, other portions can assist in providing perimeter protection for vertical openings and other prevention measures in construction environments. Another good resource is 1926 Subpart X on Stairways and Ladders.

2.11 LOSS ANALYSIS

With a sufficiently large sample of loss experience, accident problems can be readily identified without the need for floor testing. Consider a large number of similar facilities such as a chain of restaurants, some of which have terrazzo floors, some have smooth quarry tile floors, and some have abrasive quarry tile floors. To determine the degree of hazard by floor type, the first step is to identify the type of floor in each facility and track accidents by floor type and exposure.

2.11.1 Tracking Exposure

Determine the exposure basis for each floor type. In most businesses, business activity indicators can be used to quantify exposure. Restaurant operations may use transaction counts or man-hours to determine the exposure of people to fall hazards. Exposure is determined by multiplying the unit exposure times the number of units. Thus, if the exposure unit is store receipts, it is fairly easy to track the number of falls per million dollars of sales or per million man-hours.

The accident rate for each type of floor can readily reveal the extent of the fall hazard for each operation. If 9.6 falls occur per million dollars of sales on terrazzo, 7.3 falls per million dollars on smooth quarry tile, and 4.7 per million dollars on abrasive quarry tile, the degree of hazard for each floor type can be determined, and action plans for accident reduction can be developed.

2.11.2 Gathering the Data

Unless the proper information concerning the circumstances of each fall has been collected, it is unlikely that an analysis can be performed to support a rationale for a specific course of corrective action. To capture relevant data, accidents must first be well investigated.

Fall patterns normally arise from the type of hazards, the facility layout and design, and the activities of personnel. A fall-specific investigation report format may be needed to gather essential information for each event.

To determine what information is important, first select the most severe fall cases. On an insurance carriers' run, the amount paid plus reserve is a good indicator of severity, so look at the highest-cost cases. It may be necessary to reinvestigate these cases to develop an accurate profile. After reviewing enough losses to get a good picture of the patterns, a focused report format can be developed in order to prompt staff to develop the most pertinent information.

Establish a coding system to gather relevant information in a database for meaningful analysis. Information may include time of day, activity being performed by the victim, area of the facility, and condition of the floor. Be aware of multiple causation, and the difference between a cause and an injury when selecting codes.

Once the proper data is gathered and entered into the database, fall trends can be readily performed. This analysis will suggest obvious remedies and prioritize issues so that management can achieve significant improvement by the most efficient means.

2.11.3 Developing Solutions

After identifying the critical few problem areas, the next step is to develop solutions. For example, after realizing that most falls were occurring in kitchen and dining room areas, a hotel chain reduced falls by 50% by putting down epoxy concrete coatings for floors in kitchen areas, and virtually eliminated employee and guest falls in dining room areas with the use of carpeting.

Through analysis and testing, a large museum determined that the dust created from pedestrian traffic on soft stone flooring was contributing to falls when pedestrians walked from those areas into waxed wood floor galleries. Sealing the stone flooring prevented the accumulation of dust on shoe soles, thus significantly reducing the potential for falls.

EXHIBIT 2.1
FACILITY AND PARKING LOTS: HOURLY INSPECTION LOG

Facility and Parking Lots: Hourly Inspection Log

Facility Name:	Area Surveyed:

Instructions:

This log is a tool to help control slip and fall hazards.

The person conducting the inspection should initial the box after all the hazards identified during the inspection are eliminated and/or corrected.

Parking lots and sidewalks should be surveyed at least daily to identify unsafe conditions that can lead to falls.

Special emphasis should be placed on curbs, potholes, changes in walking levels, lighting, and traffic control.

The time completed and the employees' initials should be in the boxes marked 'wash' and 'wax.'

The department or facility manager should review the log daily and initial the box provided.

Reminder: 'Wet Floor' signs should be used when conditions warrant. Signs should be at least 36" high and positioned to visibly indicate the location of the spill.

Dates (show month/day below)

Time														
6 am														
7 am														
8 am														
9 am														
10 am														
11 am														
noon														
1 pm														
2 pm														
3 pm														
4 pm														
5 pm														
6 pm														
7 pm														
8 pm														
9 pm														
10 pm														
11 pm														
12 pm														
1 am														
2 am														
3 am														
4 am														
5 am														
Wash														
Wax														
Park														
Mgr														

EXHIBIT 2.2 SAMPLE SNOW REMOVAL REPORT[A]

Sample Snow Removal Report

Date:		Day of Week:		Temperature:		F C
Weather:	☐ Snow	☐ Sleet	☐ Hail	☐ Rain	☐ Cloudy	☐ Clear
Amount:		*ft inches*		Employee:		
Facility:				Location:		

Area	Direction				Treatment				Time		
	N	S	E	W	Plow	Blow	Salt	Sand	Time	am	pm
Steps, Front	☐	☐	☐	☐	☐	☐	☐	☐		☐	☐
Steps, Rear	☐	☐	☐	☐	☐	☐	☐	☐		☐	☐
Steps, Side	☐	☐	☐	☐	☐	☐	☐	☐		☐	☐
Steps, Side	☐	☐	☐	☐	☐	☐	☐	☐		☐	☐
Ramps	☐	☐	☐	☐	☐	☐	☐	☐		☐	☐
Access to Lots	☐	☐	☐	☐	☐	☐	☐	☐		☐	☐
Walkways, Front	☐	☐	☐	☐	☐	☐	☐	☐		☐	☐
Walkways, Rear	☐	☐	☐	☐	☐	☐	☐	☐		☐	☐
Walkways, Side	☐	☐	☐	☐	☐	☐	☐	☐		☐	☐
Walkways, Side	☐	☐	☐	☐	☐	☐	☐	☐		☐	☐
Other:	☐	☐	☐	☐	☐	☐	☐	☐		☐	☐
Other:	☐	☐	☐	☐	☐	☐	☐	☐		☐	☐
Other:	☐	☐	☐	☐	☐	☐	☐	☐		☐	☐
Other:	☐	☐	☐	☐	☐	☐	☐	☐		☐	☐

Employee:	Title:
Date Completed:	Time Completed: am pm
Comments	

3 Principles of Slip Resistance

3.1 INTRODUCTION

It could be argued that falls as a result of slips are the most frequent type of fall accident. In order to effectively apply assessment and measurement techniques for slip resistance, it is essential to have a working knowledge of the underlying principles of friction, factors that affect traction on walkway surfaces, and the origins of measurement instruments and related thresholds of safety. Knowledge of these principles permits informed decision making regarding appropriate methods of measuring traction, critical factors that contribute to or hamper pedestrian traction, and meaningful interpretation of slip resistance test results.

3.2 PRINCIPLES OF FRICTION

Leonardo da Vinci stated two of the three laws of measuring forces contributing to friction. The first is that the frictional force is proportional to the load (e.g., the static coefficient of friction [SCOF] is equal to the horizontal force needed to just start the object in motion, divided by the vertical force [weight] of the object, or SCOF = H/V [horizontal over vertical]. The second principle is that the coefficient of friction is independent of the area of contact. The third principle (first expressed by Coulomb) is that the friction is independent of the sliding velocity. Friction, then, depends only on the applied load. The coefficient of friction, which is the ratio of the load to the force required for movement, should be constant under all conditions. In practice, the first two laws are generally true with only about a 10% variation, but it has been recognized that friction is not independent of the sliding velocity (speed).

In 1835, A. Morin proposed that, because the force resisting the start of sliding was obviously not the same as the force required to maintain sliding, two different coefficients of friction were operating. The first is the SCOF, which is the relative force (H/V) required to start motion in a body at rest. The second coefficient is the dynamic coefficient of friction (DCOF), which is the relative force required to maintain motion in a sliding body. Generally, SCOF produces a higher number than DCOF because it takes more force to initiate a sliding motion than to keep a sliding object in motion.

Given the three laws of friction, measuring SCOF can be considered a simple procedure: place a weighed block on a surface, attach a strain gauge, and measure the "pull" (in pounds) required to move the block, divided by the weight of the block in pounds (see Figure 3.1).

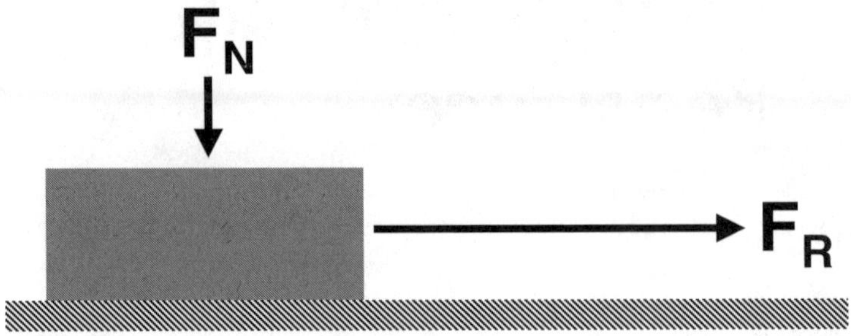

FIGURE 3.1 The classic physics definition of SCOF.

In the 1940s, it became clear that the results of this simple method of measuring SCOF did not correlate to the perception of human ambulation. A rethinking of the interrelation of friction and velocity occurred in 1939 when F. P. Bowden and L. L. Leben, physical chemists at the University of Cambridge, identified the "stick-slip" phenomenon. It was established that friction first increases with velocity and then declines. Ernest Rabinowicz puts forth a clear explanation of this phenomenon in his 1956 article in *Scientific American,* titled "Stick and Slip":

> *. . . if the slide of one surface over another slows down, friction increases. However, at extremely slow speeds the situation is reversed: as friction increases the sliding velocity also increases. The most plausible explanation seems to lie in the phenomenon called creep. All materials slowly change shape ("creep") even under moderate forces. An increase in force will increase the rate of creep.*
>
> *Thus in the case of surfaces sliding very slowly over each other, an increase in frictional force may produce a perceptible acceleration of the slide in the form of creep of one surface past the other. The limit of speed attained by the creep mechanism varies with the material, because soft materials creep faster than hard ones.*
>
> *These considerations present us with the paradoxical conclusion that there is really no such thing as a static coefficient of friction for most materials. Any frictional force applied to them will produce some creep, i.e., motion.*

3.3 SLIP RESISTANCE DEFINED

When discussing the coefficient of friction (COF) and/or slip resistance, it is essential to understand that a walkway surface does not have a COF or slip resistance in and of itself. This measure is a function of the interaction between two surfaces: the walkway surface (or surrogate) and the footwear bottom (or surrogate). When using these terms, the composition, type, and condition of both surfaces are relevant. Because slip resistance is an interaction between two variables (e.g., walkway and footwear bottom), it is essential that when evaluating one (i.e., the walkway), the other must be a constant or control material (e.g., footwear bottom surrogate material).

The term "slip resistance" is generally favored by organizations that write standards for human ambulation, instead of the term "coefficient of friction." COF measurements can be made for many reasons (e.g., ball-bearing properties), while slip resistance measurements are generally understood to be COF measurements used to assess pedestrian walkway and footwear safety.

So, whereas the classic physics type of equipment does measure SCOF as expressed in the three laws (SCOF = H/V), this system does not incorporate the host of other variables associated with human ambulation. People do not walk by sliding their feet. Additional biomechanical factors of walking have been incorporated into some tribometers that have been developed more recently. The more closely an instrument is able to emulate human ambulation, the more closely the instrument results are likely to correlate to the human perception of slipperiness.

3.4 SLIP RESISTANCE FACTORS

Four primary physical factors affect traction between the shoe and the floor surface:

1. Material and finish of the floor (controllable)
2. Footwear-bottom material and condition (generally uncontrollable, except in the workplace)
3. Environmental contaminants (controllable)
4. Gait dynamics (i.e., how an individual walks)

Whereas floor design and condition are controllable, the types of footwear worn by individuals as well as how these individuals walk usually are not. The exception to this is employee safety, especially when special footwear is needed for a given occupation or task.

In simple terms, walking is a method of locomotion in which the body weight (or center of gravity) is carried alternatively by the right and left foot. Contact with the walkway occurs in four distinct phases:

1. *Heel Strike* — the initial touch down of the footwear on the surface in which only the back edge of the heel is in contact with the walkway surface
2. *Stance* — the point at which the foot has become flat on the walkway surface
3. *Take-Off* — when only the front portion (or ball) of the foot is in contact with the walkway surface and it pushes off to move forward
4. *Swing* — when the foot is being passed forward off the ground

It is understandable (and well known) that the majority of slip and fall occurrences are the result of the heel strike phase of walking. At that point, body weight is being transferred from the trailing leg to the leading leg, which is contacting the walkway surface only by the edge of the heel.

Under low-traction conditions, the heel edge will begin to slide before an opportunity arises for the walker to make full contact with the heel, or to compensate for the slide (see Figure 3.2).

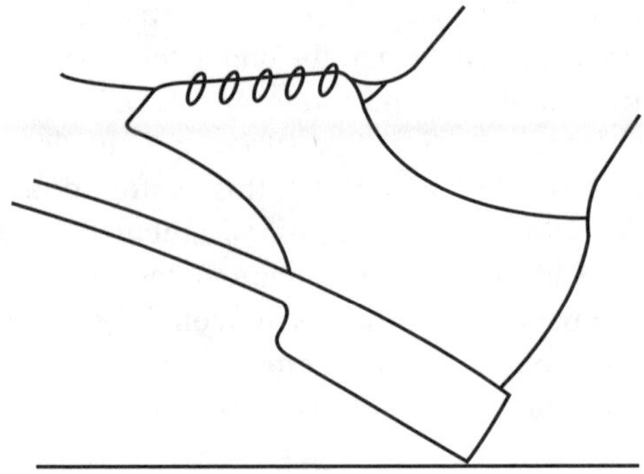

FIGURE 3.2 An illustration of the heel-strike phase of human ambulation.

3.5 SLIP RESISTANCE SCALE

The slip resistance scale ranges from a minimum of zero to a maximum of one, measured in tenths of a point. The closer the rating is to zero, the less slip resistant the surface. For example, a rating of 0.1 is considered unusually slippery, while a rating of 0.9 is considered very safe.

Studies have indicated that ice measures at about 0.20, while the minimum amount of traction needed for walking is 0.25. The often-mentioned 0.50 guideline includes a factor for safety; this factor is needed because conditions other than the walkway surface (such as footwear) could increase the hazard. Whereas the U.S. generally favors 0.50 (based on an SCOF approach), overseas, a threshold of 0.40 (based on a DCOF approach) is most often cited. These guidelines are discussed in Chapters 4 and 5.

It appears that a recommendation from Sidney James of Underwriters Laboratory to the Casualty Council of Underwriters Laboratories in 1945 was the first mention of the 0.5 threshold. This was probably based on a combination of laboratory test results using the James Machine and field experience over several years. This guideline made its way into the floor wax and floor polish industry; although no known accident statistics to support this threshold have been published.

In 1953, the Federal Trade Commission (FTC) published a set of 20 Proposed Trade Rules for the Floor Wax and Floor Polish Industry, which included the following:

> *Rule 5 – Improper Use of the Terms "Slip Resistant" (See Definitions), "Slip Retardant," Anti-slip," etc.*
>
> *Note: Subject to the development and acceptance of improved testing methods, either or both of the following tests with resultant coefficients of friction may be employed for the purpose of compliance with this rule:*
>
> *(1) A [dynamic] coefficient of friction of not less than 0.40…Sigler test…*
>
> *(2) A [static] coefficient of friction of not less than 0.5…by the test for slip resistance…by Underwriters Laboratories Inc. [James Machine]…"*

This rule and the other proposed rules were never issued as final rules.

The American Society of Testing and Materials (ASTM) Committee D21 on Wax Polishes and Related Materials was formed in 1950 and immediately began work on the slip resistance issue, considering the James and Sigler instruments. It was not until 1964, however, that tentative method D2047–64T was issued, calling for the use of the James Machine only. In 1969, ASTM D-2047 was adopted, which specified the use of the James Machine for polishes, but it contained no threshold. In 1970, the Chemical Specialties Manufacturers Association (CSMA, now the Consumer Specialty Products Association [CSPA]) adopted ASTM D-2047 with the provision that 0.5 be the threshold. In 1974, ASTM D-2047 incorporated the threshold of 0.5. For more details, see Chapter 4.

Currently, no standard or law requires that floors must have a certain level of slip resistance. Historical precedent, standards, guidelines, and case law all point to 0.5 as a reasonable threshold, however, and it is the most generally recognized and accepted value in the U.S.

3.6 SURFACE ROUGHNESS

The property of a floor that makes it slip resistant in the presence of contaminants such as water or oil is its surface roughness. Several measures are used to determine surface roughness. Two key factors for the purposes of slip resistance are the sharpness of the asperities (i.e, peaks and valleys) and the depth of asperities.

Long before instruments for measuring roughness became available, contractors increased the roughness of sidewalks, highways, and exterior stairs by broom finishing, rock-salt finishing, machine grinding, and other means. The purpose was to increase wet slip resistance without changing the composition of the base material.

3.6.1 Height or Sharpness

Some researchers cite recent studies indicating that some parameters, which are calculated purely from surface heights using roughness meters, directly correlate with the measured slip resistance. They believe that the shape of surface peaks is only one factor, and that other factors are equally important.

Others believe that measuring with roughness meters as a way of assessing slip resistance is limited because of their inability to take into account anything but the distance from high to low points on the surface. Slip resistance is as much a function of the sharpness of asperities as it is of the mean peak-to-valley distance. By experimentation, it can be demonstrated that a flat surface with pits in it (which would register a certain "roughness" with a surface comparator) performs about the same as the same surface without the pits.

Similarly, surface peaks that are rounded off from surface wear may still show a high peak-to-valley distance, but traction performance will be reduced. It is common on ramps, in fact, to be able to measure a directionality of traction. Normally, floor traffic will wear the peaks off on the high side (as would be expected in downhill traffic) so that higher traction numbers are calculated when measuring uphill than downhill.

A precision workshop using Taylor Hobson Surtronic roughness meters was conducted in 2000 by the U.K. Slip Resistance Group (see Chapter 7). Nine instruments were tested on five surface textures. One such instrument obtained results ranging from 0.5 to 1.5 on the same surface; another yielded 0.4 to 13.1 on the same surface, suggesting that roughness meters may not be as precise and sensitive as needed for the purposes of the fine measurement of roughness related to slip resistance.

Sharpness is the major contributor to slip resistance: the sharper the peaks are, the more slip resistant the surface. On a microscopic scale, all surfaces have asperities; it is these asperities that must be tall enough and sharp enough to extend upward through a contaminant to engage the shoe bottom. Therefore, it is important to select flooring materials that are sufficiently rough with durable micropeaks that will protrude through a contaminant and engage or "dig into" the shoe bottom over the life of the material.

3.6.2 Liquid Dispersion

The ability of a floor to disperse liquid quickly is greatly affected by the surface texture of the floor. Many slips occur because of the buildup of what is known as a hydrodynamic squeeze film. This is similar to what happens to a car tire when it hydroplanes on a wet road. The peak-to-valley depth also has some impact. The deeper are the asperities, the greater is the ability of the surface to channel water away from the footwear–walkway interface, which reduces the potential for hydroplaning.

3.6.3 Assessing Roughness

The two primary methods of measuring roughness are roughness gauges (most commonly the Taylor Hobson Surtronic 10) and profilometers (generally, laboratory instruments). High-powered photographic microscopes (e.g., scanning electron microscope (SEM) photomicrographs) are also used, but they are considered expensive laboratory equipment.

G. W. Harris and S. R. Shaw first published the relationship of human traction to the combination of Rtm and dynamic friction in the *Journal of Occupational Accidents* in 1988. They suggested 10 microns as a minimum for Rtm. An accompanying paper by Proctor and Coleman in the same issue quoted the 10-micron minimum.

In 1993, Proctor, in *Safety Science,* reviewed research in the field and confirmed the finding of Harris and Shaw that an Rtm of 10 microns or more is necessary to ensure the safety of pedestrians on wet walkways. In 1995, a paper by Rowland et al. at *Polymer Testing '95* reiterated the 10-micron Rtm minimum for wet walkways.

3.7 WET SURFACES

A majority of slip/fall incidents occur as a result of contact with a spot on the floor surface that is unexpectedly slippery, usually due to moisture. It is important to determine how slip resistant the surface is under dry *and* wet conditions because of pedestrian "expectation."

3.7.1 Hydroplaning

The problem of hydroplaning also exists with wet surfaces, in which the foot is momentarily supported by the film of liquid on the surface, not by the surface below. When hydroplaning occurs, the slip resistance of the surface becomes irrelevant. This phenomenon occurs most often when the liquid is very slippery (e.g., as oil) and when the application force is minimal (e.g., when the heel first touches down). Aside from good housekeeping, the best way to minimize hydroplaning is to increase the roughness of the floor surface. This measure minimizes the conditions that contribute to hydroplaning.

3.7.2 Sticktion

"Sticktion" is the name that safety professionals give to a temporary bond created between the test foot of a slip meter and the walkway surface when contact is made. Often referred to in the literature as "stick-slip," this phenomenon was well discussed by Rabinowicz as early as 1956. Sticktion creates unrealistically high slip resistance readings on wet surfaces, sometimes producing results even higher than the same surface when tested in dry conditions. The cause of sticktion is "residence time," or the delay between the time the test foot of the slip meter contacts the floor (i.e., vertical force due to gravity) and the application of the horizontal force. R. B. Hunter in his research of 1929 pointed out that, on wet surfaces, the "apparently abnormally high values of coefficients of friction under these conditions may not be due to an actual increase in friction. They may be explained on the assumption that perfect contact is made, and that a seal is formed between the wet or oily surfaces giving the effect of a partial vacuum under the shoe."

Rabinowicz (1956) explained:

> *. . . In any adhesive process the bond becomes stronger the longer it is left undisturbed. This is why the static coefficient of friction increases with time of contact. In the case of sliding surfaces, the period of contact between points on the two surfaces is, of course, longer when the surfaces slide slowly than when they move rapidly. Consequently, if the slide of one surfaced over another slows down, friction increases. This is the situation that favors stick slip. However, laboratory tests have developed the unexpected finding that at extremely slow speeds the situation is reversed: as friction increases the sliding velocity also increases.*

Examples of tribometers that can produce sticktion are the horizontal pull slip meter and the Tortus-type instruments, in which a weight is placed on the surface and is pulled (or dragged) across the floor (see Figure 3.3). Slip meters that apply horizontal and vertical forces simultaneously generate no residence time, however. As a result, they can avoid sticktion.

3.8 CLASSES OF TRIBOMETERS

The three classes of slip resistance testers are discussed next.

3.8.1 Horizontal Pull (Dragsled)

The basic principle of the horizontal pull, or dragsled, meter is the pulling of footwear or surrogate material against a walkway surface under a fixed load (or weight) at a constant speed. Some devices are manually pulled, and some are motorized. Dragsled-type meters measure friction in the classic physics sense — SCOF = H/V.

Figure 3.3 depicts the horizontal pull tribometer.

3.8.2 Pendulum

The basic principle of the pendulum class of slip resistance tester involves the calculation of energy loss as an indirect measurement of slip resistance. The pendulum is raised to a fixed height above the surface and is swung across it. As the test foot crosses the walkway, a spring presses the foot material against the surface. The rubbing of the foot on the surface results in a loss of energy due to friction determined by the reduced length of the swing.

Figure 3.4 depicts a pendulum tribometer.

3.8.3 Articulated Strut

Articulated strut tribometers are considered by many experts to be the most reliable and accurate type of slip resistance testers. These devices apply a fixed speed and angle, representing the best simulation of human ambulation of the three classes (see Figure 3.5).

3.9 HUNTER MACHINE

The Hunter Machine (see Figure 3.6) is the grandfather of all slip resistance test instruments. R. B. Hunter developed it as a result of his work under project A-22

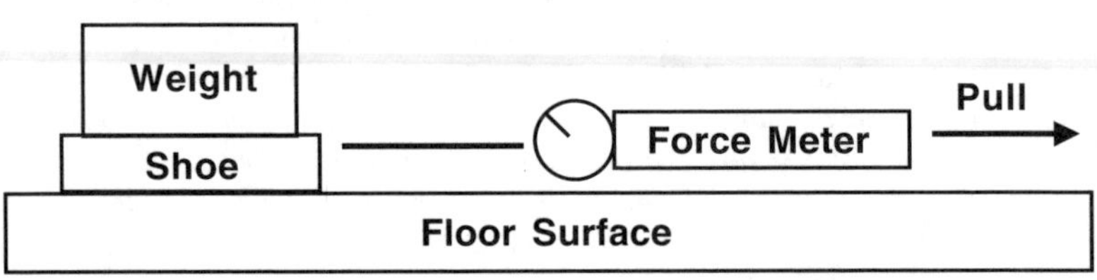

FIGURE 3.3 Horizontal pull tribometer.

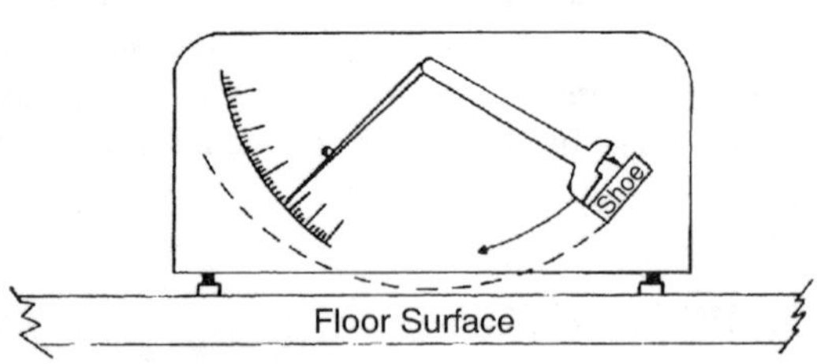

FIGURE 3.4 Pendulum tribometer.

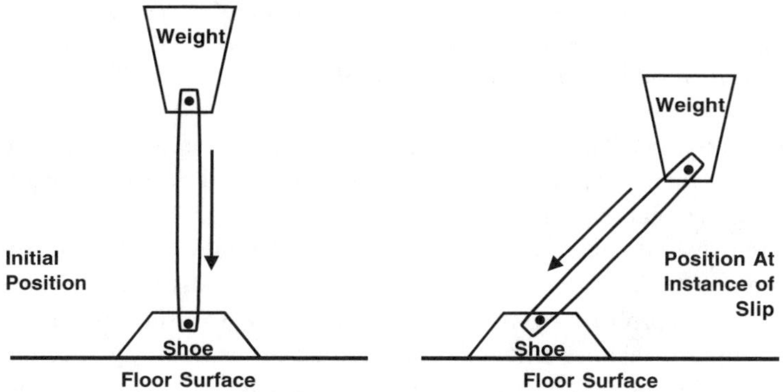

FIGURE 3.5 Articulated strut tribometer.

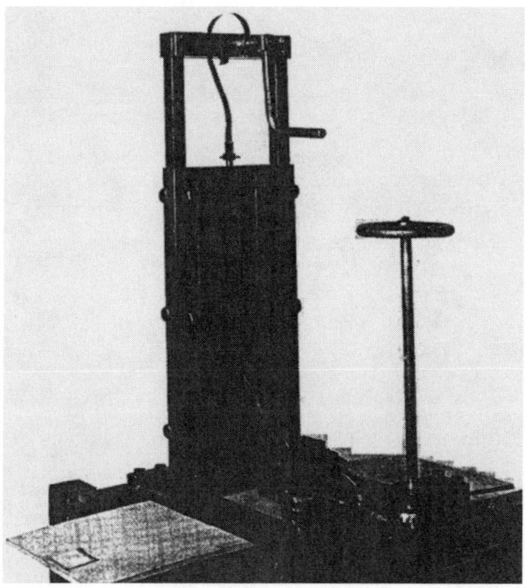

FIGURE 3.6 Hunter Machine.

of the American Standards Association (now the American National Standards Institute [ANSI]) during his research in the field from 1924 to 1929. In his 1929 article, "*A Method of Measuring Frictional Coefficients of Walk-Way Materials," in the Bureau of Standards Journal of Research,* R. B. Hunter describes the instrument:

> *It operates on an oblique thrust principle corresponding to the thrust on the shoe in walking and consists of a right-angled frame carrying a slotted 75-pound weight between two vertical bars of the frame which serve as guides to the weight. A 10-inch thrust arm is pivoted at one end near the center of gravity of the weight and at the other end through the center of area of a 3 by 3 inch shoe. The weight…is supported in the raised position by the friction of the shoe on the surface under test. By means of a screw and lug the shoe may be drawn forward by small increments, increasing*

> *the horizontal component of the force until the shoe slips on the surface, letting the weight drop…The lug carries an index which shoes the horizontal distance of the shoe from its position when the thrust arm is vertical.*

Subsequently, in 1940, the laboratories of Liberty Mutual Insurance Company developed a portable version of the Hunter Machine; however, this instrument, similar to the original, was never widely used or accepted.

Although several subsequent inventions were laboratory only devices that had an adhesion and sticktion problem, the Hunter Machine was a portable field device that overcame this problem by avoiding residence time. Considered a dynamic COF tester, the Hunter Machine dragged a test pad across a walkway specimen until a slip occurred. The literature does not indicate whether it was ever commercially produced. Photographs of the instrument are also hard to find, although a portable variant of the Hunter Machine was apparently made.

4 ASTM Standards Related to Pedestrian Safety

4.1 INTRODUCTION

The American Society for Testing and Materials (ASTM) is the most active U.S. standards-making organization in the development of slip resistance related standards. ASTM currently has eight active standards for six different slip meters. These include the build-it-yourself horizontal dynamometer pull meter method, the 1960s era horizontal pull slipmeter (HPS), the laboratory-only James Machine, and the proprietary portable inclinable articulated strut tester (PIAST) and variable incidence tribometer (VIT) devices. Some methods are only approved for specific uses. With two exceptions (polishes and bathtubs), ASTM slipmeter standards presently provide no threshold of safety. They are test methods, or steps to follow to arrive at (presumably) valid results using the specified test device.

No two slipmeters agree, even on dry surfaces, and most either have not been approved or have proven unreliable for wet testing. No known correlation exists between most of the devices. In part, this is because most of these instruments have their own set of biases and operator variability issues, and because friction is a property of the system used to measure it.

4.2 ASTM INTERNATIONAL (FORMERLY AMERICAN SOCIETY FOR TESTING AND MATERIALS)

Organized in 1898, ASTM is one of the largest voluntary standards development organizations in the world. ASTM is a nonprofit organization with more than 32,000 members from more than 100 countries. Due to this international scope, the organization was renamed ASTM International in 2001 (http://www.astm.org).

ASTM develops standards in 130 areas, covering subjects such as metals, paints, plastics, textiles, construction, energy, the environment, consumer products, medical devices, electronics, and many others. More than 10,000 ASTM standards are published annually, all of which are "full consensus" documents (see Chapter 8 appendix).

Standards development work begins when members of a committee identify a need, or other interested parties approach the committee. Task group members prepare a draft standard, which is reviewed by its parent subcommittee through a letter ballot. After the subcommittee approves the document, it is submitted concurrently to the main committee and the Society. All members are provided an opportunity to vote on each standard. All negative votes cast during the balloting process, which must include a written explanation of the voters' objections, must be fully considered before the document can be submitted to the next level in the process. Final approval of a standard depends on concurrence by the ASTM Committee on Standards that proper procedures were followed and due process was afforded.

The number of voting producers on a committee cannot exceed the combined number of voting nonproducers (i.e., users, ultimate consumers, and those having general interest); this is intended to prevent any one party from being able to dominate the process. If a member feels the standards development process has been unfair, appeal options are available within the Society.

Note: ASTM standards cited herein are subject to reapproval and revision. As such, it is important to consult the most current edition of these standards.

4.3 TECHNICAL COMMITTEE ASTM F-13

In the 1970s, ASTM Committee E-17 Skid Resistance included subcommittee E17.26 Methods of Measuring Pedestrian Friction, which did a substantial amount of research into slip resistance measurement, including a symposium on Pedestrian Friction in 1977 (and the subsequent Special Technical Publication known as STP 649).

Long since disbanded, the work of subcommittee E17.26 continued with ASTM Committee F-13. The title of the ASTM F-13 technical committee was Safety and Traction for Footwear. Established in 1973 and originally created to develop standards relating only to footwear, its name was a bit misleading because its scope also included safety and traction for walkway surfaces, as well as practices related to the prevention of slips and falls. The committee changed its name in February 2003 to Pedestrian/Walkway Safety and Footwear to more closely align it with the scope:

> *... to develop consensus standard test methods, guidelines, practices, definitions, criteria, and nomenclature for pedestrian safety, for the fit and function of footwear in relation to interfaces, walking surfaces and devices used for the evaluation of pedestrian traction.*

F-13, one of ASTM's larger committees at approximately 300 members, is divided into several subcommittees, one of which is F13.10 Traction, which has jurisdiction over all tribometer standards. The F-13 standard is currently applied to five tribometers.

4.4 F489 STANDARD TEST METHOD FOR USING A JAMES MACHINE

Sidney James of Underwriters Laboratories developed one of the earliest slipmeters, the James Machine, in the 1940s. The James Machine is a laboratory apparatus for dry testing only (Figure 4.1). As an articulated strut class of tribometer, the James Machine applies a known constant vertical to a test pad (i.e., a leather pad when testing flooring materials), and then applies an increasing lateral force until a slip occurs. A more detailed description follows.

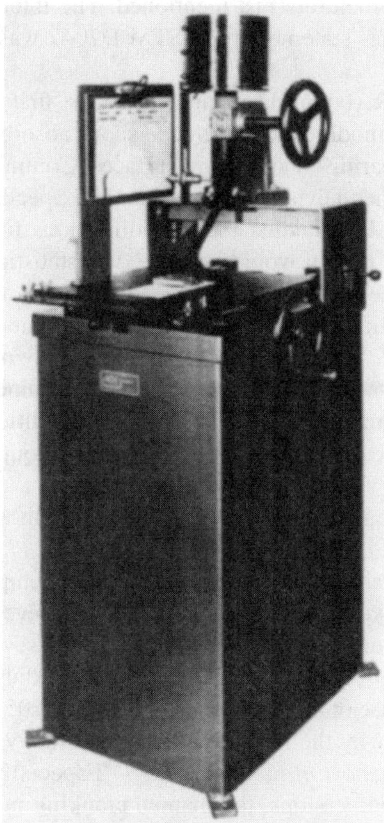

FIGURE 4.1 The manually propelled version of the James Machine.

Similar to the Hunter Machine, the test foot is a 3 in. x 3 in. piece of standard leather secured to a flat steel plate. The plate is hinged to an articulated strut 10 in. long. A 75 to 80-lb weight is vertically and downwardly applied to the strut. The hand wheel is released, and the load is transmitted to the test foot through the strut. The test foot remains in stationary contact with the test surface. The angle of inclination of the strut to the vertical is increased gradually, until it reaches the value at which the test foot slips on the test surface. The test foot carries a pointer that indicates the coefficient of friction (COF) at the point of slip on a scale attached to the machine's frame.

The James Machine functions in a way similar to a dragsled with one notable difference: The James Machine has a method for applying the friction force in an operator-insensitive manner.

The original versions of the James Machine had a hand-driven transport table. These machines were produced by a number of manufacturers, including TMI, Gardner, and Timken. These are the machines illustrated in the drawings in ASTM D2047 and F489.

By the early 1950s, some of the owners of these machines modified them for motorized test table transport, and motorized machines were made commercially available from the manufacturers just mentioned. The interlaboratory study for the original precision and bias statement for ASTM D2047 was developed with this set of machines.

In the early 1990s, R. Jablonski manufactured the first physical modification of the James Machine. The modifications included shock absorbers to cushion the falling weight, and improved bearings and bearing surfaces. Committee D21.06 (Slip Resistance) and the Maintenance Division of the Chemical Specialty Manufacturers Association (CSMA, now CSPA) studied these modifications for 3 years in order to be certain that the modified design would produce data statistically consistent with that of the other extant James Machines. Reportedly, it did, with a higher degree of repeatability and reproducibility (i.e., narrower error limits), so it was accepted as being a "James Machine" for use in D2047; however, only nine production machines were made before Professor Jablonski withdrew his machine from the market.

In 1997, the Michelmann Corporation developed additional modifications: computer interface, electronic self-diagnosis, and digital readout, along with the standard CSPA paper charts.

The challenges facing users of the James Machine include:

- The instrument has a several inherent biases, which prompted users of this instrument to make modifications in order to achieve good repeatability on a single instrument and good correlation between several similar machines.
- The device needs continuous maintenance and adjustment, in part due to the required release of a heavy weight. ASTM D6205 (see Section 4.11.1.1) lists ten reasons why the instrument can yield faulty results, including:
  - *Irregular transport of the test table* — Especially in the case of manually propelled versions, the manual cranking must be done smoothly and uniformly for accurate readings.
  - *Improper rate of transport of test table* — The rate of travel is a key factor in obtaining valid results. In the case of manually propelled versions, this is difficult to judge subjectively.
  - Wear or binding of bearings, pivots, and other components.
  - *Flat and levelness of test table* — No specified method is used for evaluating flatness.
  - Excessive movement in the strut rack gear.
  - Warped or out-of-line back plate, chart board, strut arm, or strut rack gear, often caused by improper maintenance or storage, or by the result of the impact of the heave weight applied.

As far back as 1966, Underwriters Laboratory recognized these variables and cautioned the adoption and widespread use of the James Machine:

- Due to the heavy weight applied, non-smooth surfaces (i.e., textured, rough) cannot be evaluated because the roughness can result in damage to the test foot material.
- As a laboratory-based machine, it can only be used on flooring material samples, not in-service floors (see Section 4.11.1.1 on "D2047").

- Because the device is subject to "sticktion" (see Chapter 3), and it specifies the use of leather (leather's properties change when wet, delivering overly optimistic readings), this device can only be used to test dry surfaces.
- Meaningful precision and bias testing to validate repeatability and reproducibility have yet to be conducted as of this writing. Although both James Machine Standards (F489 and D2047) tacitly include four different versions of the machine, no known works have been published about the correlation of results to each other.

In addition to the manually operated original, a hydraulically operated version, known as the Jablonsky low-friction model, is available (currently in production by Quadra Corporation and sells for about $15,000) as well as the Michelman computerized version (see Figure 4.2 and http://www.performanceadditives.com/jamz-test.htm), which currently sells for about $23,000. In addition, machine shop drawings of the apparatus are available from the CSPA, permitting any organization to build the original manually propelled version.

Dr. Robert Brungraber, while at Bucknell University (Lewisburg, PA), had the following observation regarding other unresolved concerns with this test apparatus (Brungraber et al., 1992):

> *… the tangent of the angle of inclination of the articulated strut is equal to the static coefficient of friction only if both the shoe and the articulated strut are weightless.… It is my opinion that either James never analyzed his device or else he assumed that his use of an 85-pound superimposed weight made the weights of his shoe and strut negligible. I have never analyzed the James Machine but the ones that I have seen use rather heavy steel struts and shoes, that may very well not be negligible. James also appears to have ignored any friction losses in his device which I also believe to be unwarranted.*

For more information on the use of the James Machine for the measurement of walkway-related materials, see ASTM D21 and D2047 in Sections 4.11.1 and 4.11.1.1, respectively. The research report of the precision workshop conducted to validate this test method can be obtained from ASTM for a nominal fee.

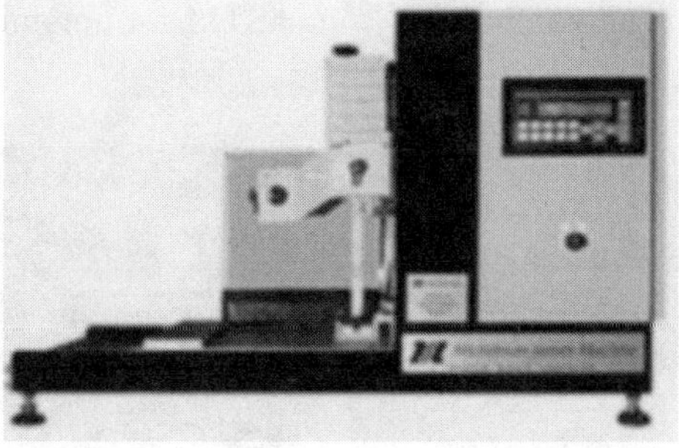

FIGURE 4.2 The Michelman computerized version of the James Machine.

4.5 F609 STANDARD TEST METHOD FOR USING A HORIZONTAL PULL SLIPMETER (HPS)

The HPS, approved for dry testing only, was developed by Charles Irvine in 1965, when he was working for Liberty Mutual Insurance Company. The basic principle of the HPS, a dragsled class of slipmeter, is the pulling of footwear or surrogate material against a walkway surface under a fixed load at a constant velocity. The HPS consists of a 6-lb weight onto which is attached a force gauge with a slip index meter. This component is attached to a nylon string and pulled by a capstan-headed motor. As the weight/meter is pulled across the walkway surface, a direct reading from the meter can be obtained (Figure 4.3).

Aside from the problem of "sticktion," which makes this device unreliable on wet surfaces, other concerns include:

- The use of a spring combined with the analog indicator makes it difficult to obtain a definitive reading.
- The lack of structure between the motor and the meter/weight (a nylon string) results in potential operator variances in the application of lateral forces.
- It is difficult to obtain valid readings on interlocking (i.e., tiled) surfaces because the sensors on the HPS are so small that they can become caught or influenced by these surface irregularities. Thus, the HPS is best suited to linoleum and other uniform resilient floor surfaces (Figure 4.4).

Although certain devices are based on similar dragsled technology, the only ASTM-approved versions of the HPS (manufactured by Whitely Industries and Creativity Inc.) were no longer commercially available until recently. Two manufacturers (Trusty-Step Products and C.S.C. Force Measurement) have begun producing the HPS. The Trusty-Step instrument (TSI-9010 Slipmeter, http://www.trusty-step.com) currently sells for $995. Although it is similar to the ASTM HPS, it does not appear to meet all the specifications of that test method — most notably, the use of a specific Chatillon force gauge.

As of 2002, work was under way by a task group of ASTM F13 to update this standard. The original research report of the precision workshop conducted to validate this test method can be obtained from ASTM for a nominal fee.

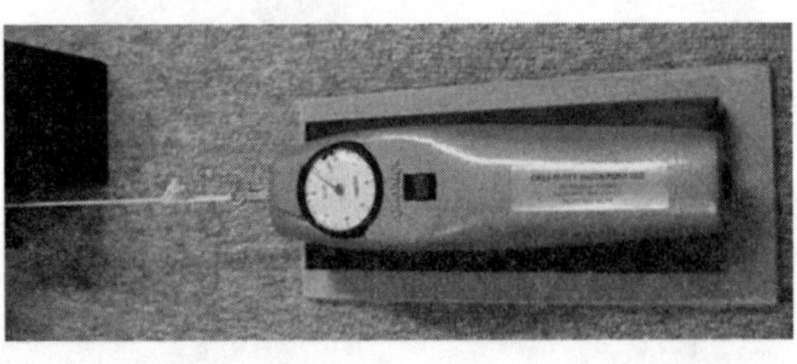

FIGURE 4.3 The Whitely Industries version of the ASTM horizontal pull slipmeter.

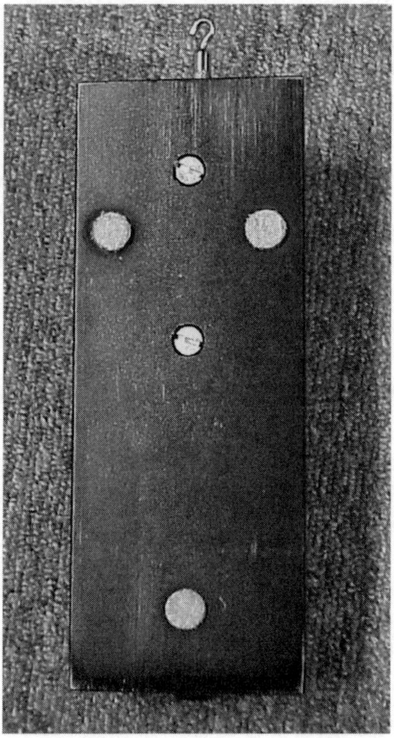

FIGURE 4.4 The underside of the HPS, showing three ½-in. circular test pads.

4.6 F1678 STANDARD TEST METHOD FOR USING A PORTABLE ARTICULATED STRUT SLIP TESTER (PAST)

While working for the National Bureau of Standards (NBS), which is now known as the National Institute for Standards and Testing, Dr. Brungraber developed the NBS-Brungraber in the 1970s (Brungraber, 1977). This slip tester was originally known as the "NBS Standard Static COF Tester" and, later, as the Mark I slip tester. The NBS-Brungraber (or Mark I) is approved for dry testing only as a PAST. Similar in principle to the James Machine, the Mark I is also an articulated strut instrument approved only for dry testing (Figure 4.5). However, it is a portable device that can test actual floors; it also uses a graduated rod that provides a direct reading from the device.

A 10-lb weight is attached to the upper end of a pair of vertical rods, which are free to move through linear ball bushings in the carriage. The carriage is also free to move horizontally along a second pair of rods under the control of a spring. Connecting the lower ends of the vertical rods and the test foot is a 10-in. shaft, hinged at both ends. The test foot (3 in. × 3 in. — the same dimensions as the James Machine test foot) is generally made of standard leather.

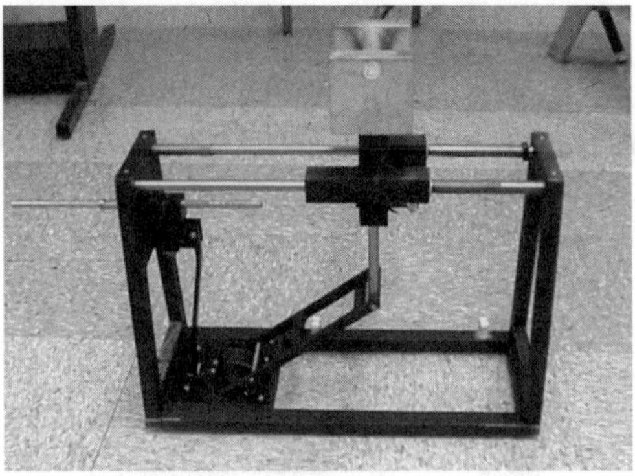

FIGURE 4.5 The NBS-Brungraber, or Mark I, PAST.

The tester is placed with the test foot in contact with the walkway surface and the carriage to the left end of the horizontal rods, so that the shaft is vertical and the test foot is subjected only to a vertical force. As the carriage moves to the right under the control of the spring, the inclination of the shaft increases, resulting in an increasing lateral force on the test foot. When this force exceeds the vertical force times the static COF, a slip occurs, which activates a trigger mechanism that blocks further motion of an indicator rod that has been drawn along by the carriage by means of a weak magnetic force (Figure 4.6).

Some calculation is required to convert this to a slip resistance measurement. Because the test foot rests on the walkway surface, the instrument is still subject to "sticktion," making it inappropriate for wet testing.

The U.S. Government patented the NBS-Brungraber (U.S. Patent No. 3,975,940; issued August 24, 1976). Although it is available for license to any U.S. entity, the only producer of the instrument has been Slip Test Inc., owned and operated by Dr.

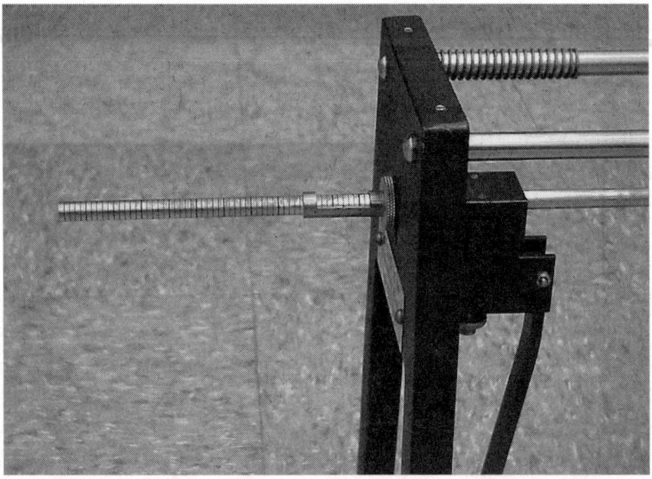

FIGURE 4.6 The NBS-Brungraber graduated rod, from which readings are obtained.

Brungraber. Although still in use (see Section 4.11.3.1 on "F462"), only about 100 units were ever sold, and Slip Test has indicated that it no longer manufactures the instrument. The test method currently does not contains a precision statement. Dr. Brungraber's next invention, the Mark II, has gained wider acceptance.

4.7 F1677 STANDARD TEST METHOD FOR USING A PORTABLE INCLINABLE ARTICULATED STRUT SLIP TESTER (PIAST)

In the 1980s, subsequent to the development of the Mark I device, Dr. Brungraber invented the Mark II. The Brungraber Mark II is approved for dry and wet testing as a PIAST. A gravity-based articulated strut device designed to avoid the "sticktion" problem, the Mark II enables users to meter wet surfaces. It does so by eliminating the residence time (or time delay) between the application of the vertical and horizontal forces (Figure 4.7).

Similar to the Mark I, the Mark II is a portable device fitted with a 3 in. × 3 in. test foot. It uses a 10-lb weight on an inclinable frame, with a test pad of Neolite Test Liner suspended just above the walkway surface. Each time the angle is set to a more horizontal position, the weight is released until a slip occurs. The slip resistance reading can be taken directly from the instrument.

Due to its size and weight, as well as the dimensions of the test pad, the Mark II is difficult to set up and operate on stairs. Because of its reliance on gravity for operation, it is unsuitable for measuring ramps in either the downhill or uphill direction. Instead, the Mark II must be used across the direction of travel.

In addition, the very low slip resistance readings obtained in wet tests appear to be the result of the flat position of the test foot at initial contact, trapping water between the foot and the walkway surface. This creates a hydroplaning effect (see Figure 4.8).

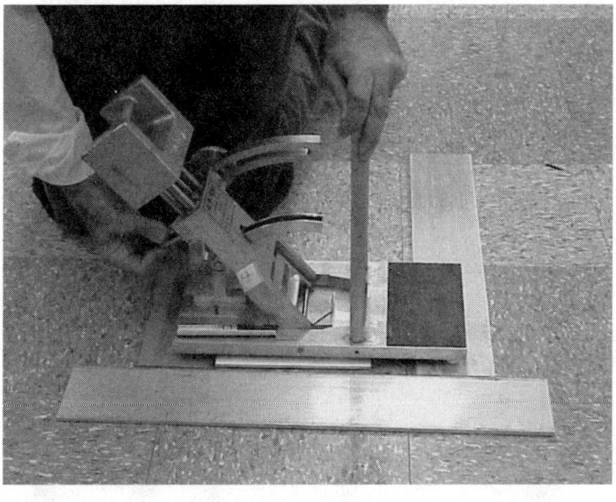

FIGURE 4.7 The Mark II PIAST.

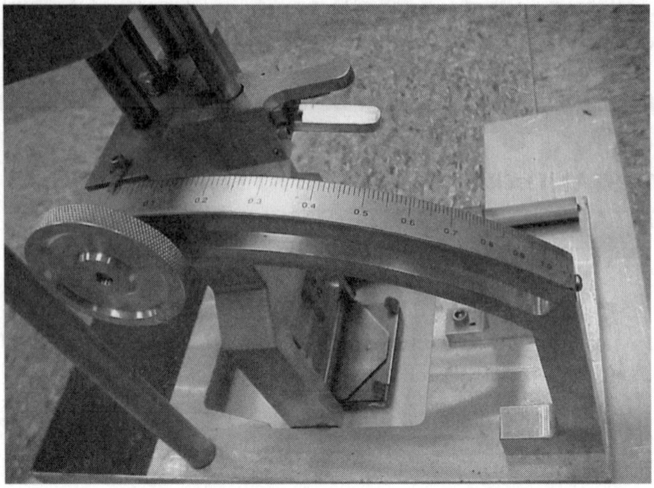

FIGURE 4.8 A direct reading of slip resistance can be obtained from the PIAST's graduated protractor.

Independent studies by several researchers (Fleisher et al., 2003; Grieser et al., 2002; Flynn and Underwood, 2000) clearly demonstrate that this effect can be overcome by using a grooved test foot on the PIAST, in order to permit a path for the displaced water. Although more study is needed to optimize the specific design (i.e., depth, width, configuration of grooves, directionality), using a grooved test foot on the PIAST also closely aligns results with that of the variable incidence tribometer (VIT). Averaged test results showed that the use of the grooved test feet on both instruments brought the readings of these devices closer to each other; using the grooved test foot, the readings generated by the PIAST and VIT were not significantly different.

Work is currently under way in F13 to provide a precision statement. The work includes ruggedness testing and a planned interlaboratory study.

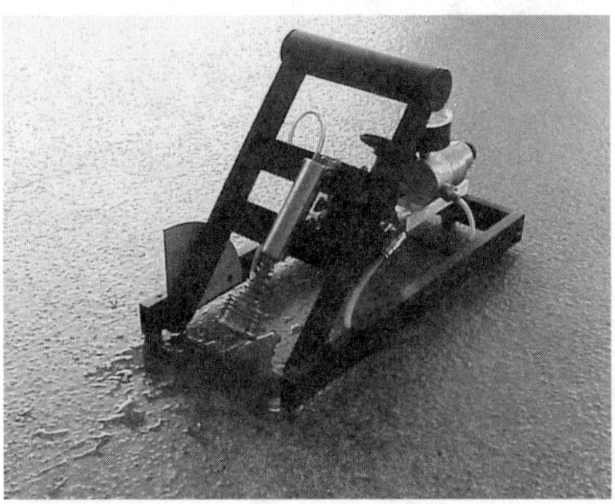

FIGURE 4.9 The English XL VIT.

The Mark II is still under patent by Dr. Brungraber's company, Slip Test Inc. (1900 Fourth Avenue, Spring Lake, NJ 07762), which is also the only manufacturer. Two applicable patents exist: U.S. Patent No. 4,759,209 (issued July 26, 1988) and U.S. Patent No. 4,798,080 (issued January 17, 1989). Currently, the Mark II can be purchased for $4000.

4.8 F1679 STANDARD TEST METHOD FOR USING A VARIABLE INCIDENCE TRIBOMETER (VIT)

In the early 1990s, William English developed the English XL™, an articulated strut device similar in principle to the Mark II. The English XL is approved for dry and wet testing as a VIT. The English XL does not rely on gravity, but is powered by a small carbon dioxide cartridge at a set pressure (Figure 4.10).

The instrument is an aluminum frame onto which is attached a hinged aluminum mast. At the base of the mast is a spring and joint assembly onto which is attached a circular test foot with a diameter of 1.25 in. The angle of the mast can be adjusted by a hand wheel from vertical 90° to 45°. The pneumatic mast is powered by a carbon-dioxide cartridge, under high pressure, through a control valve that actuates the cylinder until a slip occurs. The slip index can be read directly from the protractor mounted on the instrument. Although the standard recommends the use of Neolite Test Liner for floor testing (see Section 4.9.2), any material can be mounted on the test foot.

The instrument has several features that make it suitable for field testing:

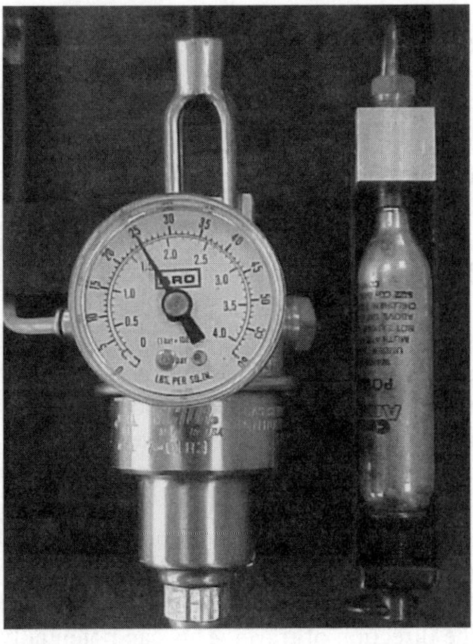

FIGURE 4.10 Using the regulator gauge, pressure is set at ±25 PSI.

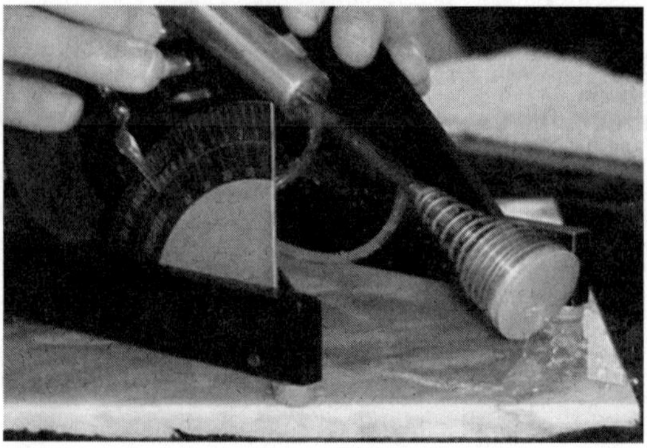

FIGURE 4.11 The VIT slipping on wet marble tile.

- The test foot cylinder contacts the walkway surface in a heel-first attitude of contact.
- The velocity of contact is consistent with strobe flash experiments of heel contact speed (Perkins, 1978).
- Whereas some researchers have suggested that the small dimensions of the test foot make the instrument inappropriate for testing of highly textured or profiled surfaces, the size of the test foot is similar to the area of heel contact in human walking.
- The compressed gas delivers a uniform force and permits metering of inclined surfaces such as ramps unhampered by the impact of gravity activation.
- Similar to the PIAST, the application of vertical and horizontal forces is simultaneous, thus avoiding residence time and permitting reliable wet test results (Figure 4.11).

In a thorough study by Powers et al. in 1999, the PIAST and VIT demonstrated remarkably low bias and good repeatability. Work by Chang and Leamon (1997) reported that the PIAST and VIT were both capable of distinguishing surface roughness on wet quarry tile. To date, F1679 is the only ASTM slip resistance test method that has undergone ruggedness testing, a procedure to measure the influence of variables on test results.

In addition, several ASTM workshops have generated much data demonstrating the reliability and consistency of the VIT. Two studies done for the revision of the Occupational Safety and Health Administration (OSHA) Steel Erection Standard bear out the correlation of the instrument's output to the human perception of walking by comparing how VIT and walkers independently rank sets of materials of various degrees of slip resistance (see http://www.cdc.gov/niosh/elcosh/docs/d0100/d000037/d000037.html). Also see the OSHA report on slip resistance for structural steel in Exhibit 4.1.

Although the VIT is capable of metering steps, the stair fixture orients the instrument opposite the direction of travel. This can potentially lead to higher-than-expected results due to the lesser amount of wear from this direction.

In addition to ruggedness testing, four ASTM-sponsored interlaboratory studies have been conducted, and a final precision statement is near completion as of this writing. A copy of the four associated research reports on these precision workshops, as well as the research report on ruggedness testing, can be obtained from ASTM for a nominal fee.

The VIT is currently still under patent (U.S. Patent No. 5,259,236; issued November 3, 1993), and the only manufacturer is William English Inc. It is available for purchase at http://www.englishxl.com for $3200 as of this writing.

4.9 TEST PAD MATERIAL

A number of slip resistance test devices (or tribometers) are available. We begin by discussing the debate on the use of test pad material for all test devices. Test pad material is the surface used on slip resistance testers that makes contact with the floor surface to obtain the slip resistance measurement. Appropriate test pad material is essential to accurate, reliable, and valid baseline readings. Of the variety of test pad materials used, only Neolite Test Liner and leather have gained wide acceptance in the U.S.

4.9.1 LEATHER

Prior to the use of Neolite, leather was the primary material used as a representative footwear bottom material. "Standard" leather is still used, which is government specification KK-L-165 Revision C(2) — Leather, Cattlehide, Vegetable Tanned and Chrome Retanned, Impregnated, and Soles, initially developed in May 1969 and amended June 1976 (see http://www.fss.gsa.gov/pub/fedspecs/sort1e.cfm).

However, many concerns arise when using leather as a constant in slip resistance testing. R. B. Hunter recognized most of these concerns in his research of 1929:

- No matter how "standardized" you try to make it, leather is not a homogenous material. In fact, being an organic substance, each piece of leather could be considered a unique material.
- It has different properties at different levels of thickness. Sanding of leather often results in a material with frictional properties different from the presanding surface.
- Leather is highly absorbent and highly sensitive to humidity. Once used for wet testing, its properties are permanently altered. This means that once leather material has been used in a wet test, it is no longer useful for dry testing.
- Leather is also not representative of heel material. Most heels are of a synthetic compound. Essentially, slips occur more on the rubber heels of leather-soled shoes.
- Leather can react differently depending on how worn the material has become. Because it reacts in a way unique to all other types of materials, it is only of value as a test material when it can be reasonably expected that most or all individuals in the area will be wearing leather soles.

Leather conforming to this Federal Specification KK-L-165C (Type 1, Class 6) is, as of this writing, only known to be available through Parsons Tanning Co. (333 Skokie Blvd, Suite 105, Northbrook, IL 60062).

4.9.2 Neolite® Test Liner

In the early 1990s, ASTM Technical Committee F13.10 began a study to identify a more suitable material than leather for walkway surface slip resistance testing. It was found that the best available material was a test grade of Neolite, originally developed, patented, and trademarked by the Goodyear Tire & Rubber Company. It is now specified by several ASTM test methods.

Despite protests to the contrary, this type of Neolite was, at one time, used by the footwear industry as a heel material. Documents from the U.S. Trademark Electronic Search System (TESS) verify that Goodyear registered this material in 1953 as "soles and heels composed of an elastomer and a resin."

Neolite is the original styrene-butadiene rubber (SBR), of which many varieties are routinely used as footwear bottom material. Under the trade name Neolite, it was sold in sheet form and die-cut to sole shapes for adhesive attachment. Its special properties were that it had flexibility and adequate wear resistance in thin substances, and felt and behaved underfoot much like leather, not like rubber. Soling of this kind has now become widely known and used, and is often referred to as resin-rubber (see http://www.cityintl.com/footwear/glossaryS-Z.htm).

To date, no more suitable material for floor friction testing has been identified for the following reasons:

- It is generic and durable substance. The characteristics of the material do not change under normal conditions, regardless of wear or moisture.
- The special test grade (or scientific grade) of Neolite Test Liner used is manufactured with specific quality controls regarding hardness and consistency of physical properties. Neolite Test Liner is manufactured to meet the now withdrawn ASTM C1028-15.02 Standard for Neolite. It is also made to a specific recipe and tested for consistency of physical properties according to a former Rubber Manufacturers' Association (RMA) specification HS-3 for use as a friction pad material, specifying shore hardness of 93–96, specific gravity of 1.25 ± 0.02, and $^1/_8$-in. thickness.
- It is stable over time.
- Its traction properties are in the median range of commonly used shoe bottom materials.
- It has been proven reliable and repeatable over many years in service as a friction pad material, and as the material of choice for the Horizontal Pull Dynamometer Pullmeter (C1028), the HPS, the PIAST, and the VIT (Flynn and Underwood, 2000). It was the material of choice by the National Bureau of Standards (now the National Institute of Standards and Technology) in its studies on the use of tribometers on wet surfaces.

The thickness of Neolite can vary (1/8 in. or 1/4 in.). Studies indicate that the results of the VIT are not dependent on the thickness of the test foot, primarily because it is a constant-velocity device being driven by gas pressure. The PIAST may show differences because it is an acceleration device.

The ASTM Board of Directors Task Group on Slip Resistance studied various recipes for (see Section 4.12), in attempts to optimize the consistency and design of this material for test purposes.

Currently, Neolite Test Liner is manufactured and supplied primarily through Smithers Scientific Services, Inc. (425 W. Market Street, Akron, OH, 44303-2099), although most any manufacturer of footwear bottom material can produce it. The consensus of many slip resistance experts is that Neolite Test Liner is the best material currently available material for testing of floor surfaces to establish slip resistance.

4.9.3 Rubbers and Other Footwear Materials

A variety of rubber compounds have been proposed (and used) as a friction pad material. In most cases, these have been in relation to overseas test methods such as the pendulum tester and the Tortus et al. (see Chapter 8 — Overseas Slip Resistance Standards).

Most rubbers have a curing period during which their properties are unstable. They also have a finite shelf life, after which their properties relating to slip resistance change again. In addition, it is difficult to locate the source of a consistent, long-term formulation. Thus, it is somewhat impractical to use most of these types of materials.

Many rubbers are at the high end of slip resistance materials currently in use for footwear, and can provide overly optimistic readings when assessing the slip resistance of flooring materials. In contrast, neoprene rubber, a specification of some U.S. Government shoes, provides low traction on lubricated surfaces. The impact of wear on rubbers is also another variable.

4.9.3.1 Neoprene

Neoprene is a synthetic rubber specified in some government shoe specifications and as test pad material in some government traction specifications. It is poor friction material for slip resistance testers because it has proven unrealistically slippery on lubricated (i.e., wet) surfaces. For this reason, neoprene is rarely used today.

4.9.3.2 4S

Rubber and Plastics Research Association (RAPRA, a European consultancy) 4S (Standard Shoe Sole Simulating) Rubber gives artificially high readings, is not consistently produced, and is costly. Although it is used for some tribometers overseas, it has not gained a significant following in the U.S.

4.9.3.3 TRRL

RAPRA also promotes TRRL rubber (Transport and Roads Research Laboratory, U.K.) for pendulum testers, which is considered well suited for assessing and comparing very rough surfaces, such as road surfaces; however, this same quality makes it a poor choice for making finer discriminations on smooth or moderate rough flooring materials. In fact, studies have indicated that TRRL rubber consistently yields slip resistance results 20 points higher (more optimistically) than RAPRA 4S.

4.9.4 Actual Footwear Bottoms

It is a common misconception that material from the actual footwear from the claimant should be used as the test pad material in accident investigations. It is clear, however, that this would not provide an objective measurement of slip resistance, since the type of material and its wear/condition significantly affects the results of the readings.

In essence, it would be difficult to determine whether the floor surface or the sole of the footwear was primarily responsible for the slip. It is essential that a consistent material must be used in order to make meaningful comparisons between floor surface readings.

4.10 OTHER ASTM F13 STANDARDS

In accordance with its scope, ASTM F13 is also responsible for developing standards relating to footwear and walkway surfaces.

4.10.1 ASTM F695

ASTM F695 is the *Standard Practice for the Evaluation Test Data Obtained by Using the HPS or the James Machine for Measurement of Static Slip Resistance of Footwear Sole, Heel, or Related Materials.*

Under the jurisdiction of F13.50 (Walkway Surface Practices subcommittee of F13), this document provides a method for a comparative ranking of test results performed using test methods in F489 and F609.

4.10.2 ASTM F1240

ASTM F1240 is a *Guide for Categorizing Results of Footwear Slip Resistance Measurements on Walkway Surfaces with an Interface of Various Foreign Substances.*

Also under F13.50, the purpose of this standard is to assist in selecting appropriate footwear in areas where foreign materials can contribute to slips and falls. Due to the similarity of F1240 with F695 (see Section 4.10.1), there are plans to combine these into a single document in the near future.

In 2002, work was completed by a task group of ASTM F13 to update this standard and combine it with F695.

4.10.3 ASTM F1637

ASTM F1637-95 is the *Practice for Safe Walking Surfaces* standard.

This standard addresses common walking surface defects and design considerations, including where slip resistant surfaces should be provided. This document is the responsibility of F13.50.

4.10.4 ASTM F1646

ASTM F1646 is the standard for *Terminology Relating to Safety and Traction for Footwear.*

A document of F13.91 (the terminology subcommittee of F13), this standard defines commonly used terms relating to slip resistance and footwear.

4.10.5 ASTM F1646

ASTM F1646 is *the Standard Guide for Composing Walkway Surface Evaluation and Incident Report Forms for Slips, Stumbles, Trips and Falls.*

Under the jurisdiction of F13.30 (the consumers subcommittee of F13), this guide provides guidance in recording and evaluating the conditions of walkway surfaces, including components such as ramps and stairs, that may present a hazard or an exposure to slip, stumble, or trip.

4.10.6 ASTM F1646

ASTM F1646 is the *Standard Guide for Selection of Certain Walkway Surfaces When Considering Footwear Traction.*

Under the jurisdiction of F13.50, this guide is intended to help when selecting walkway surfaces where the presence of foreign materials may increase the potential for a slip or fall.

4.10.7 ASTM F2048

ASTM F2048 is the *Standard Practice for Reporting Slip Resistance Test Results.*

First published in 2000, this F13.10 standard provides guidance on how to document the results of slip resistance testing. F2048 includes a sample format for collecting this information.

4.11 OTHER ASTM COMMITTEES WITH PEDESTRIAN TRACTION ACTIVITIES

Other standards relating to the measurement of pedestrian slip resistance are the responsibility of other ASTM committees, although these are more focused on test methods intended to validate the merchantability of lines of products instead of evaluation of in service walkway surfaces. Except for C1028, each of these specify devices for which there is also an ASTM F13 standard.

4.11.1 Committee D21 Polishes

Formed in 1950, D21 is responsible for 44 standards for characteristics and performance of raw materials, physical and chemical testing, performance and specifications relating to polishes. The committee scope states that D21 is concerned primarily with floor, furniture, and automotive polishes. Subcommittee D21.06 Slip Resistance publishes three standards — D2047, D4103, and D6205— which relate to testing using the James Machine.

4.11.1.1 D2047

D2047 is the *Standard Test Method for Static Coefficient of Friction of Polish-Coated Floor Surfaces as Measured by the James Machine* (under the jurisdiction of technical committee D21 Polishes).

D2047 was the first ASTM standard referring to the James Machine. One of the first orders of business of D21,when it was formed in 1950, was the topic of slip resistance. In 1964, tentative method ASTM D2047-64T was issued without a threshold specification; it became a standard in 1969. It was not until 1974 that the threshold of 0.5 was added.

D2047 and F462 (see Section 4.11.3.1) are the only ASTM test methods that currently include a threshold upon which to base a quantitative assessment of slip resistance. Related to this standard are:

- D4103-90 (1995), *Standard Practice for Preparation of Substrate Surfaces for Coefficient of Friction Testing,* which addresses the process of preparing official vinyl composition tile (OVCT) and wood panels for use in tests to measure the COF
- D6205 (1998), *Standard Practice for Calibration of the James Static Coefficient of Friction Machine,* which provides guidance on determining if the test instrument is mechanically calibrated and properly aligned

Correlation of the James Machine to actual usage is limited to several optimal conditions. These assumptions essentially involve unencumbered walking at an average pace of 3 m.p.h. on well-maintained level surfaces, free of gross debris or contamination of any type (e.g., liquid, grit). Despite its shortcomings, this instrument under D2047 continues to be used to validate the merchantability of new flooring materials and treatments.

An extensive discussion of the pitfalls of using this apparatus is discussed in Section 4.4 on ASTM F489. Although the proponents of this test method cite research done to establish a correlation between a James Machine reading of 0.5 and the human perception of a slip resistant surface, it is important to remember that the James Machine can only test flooring materials, not actual floors. Once flooring material measured by the James Machine is placed in service its properties are immediately altered by such factors as wear, contaminants, and cleaning. Any such correlations between the material in pristine condition and those subject to a variety of other unaccounted variables are at best questionable. In addition, work dating back as far as 1972 indicated that several manufacturers of polish indicated that their least slip resistant products obtained the highest James Machine COF readings. The author does not know of any published accident statistics or peer-reviewed research that support this threshold. As discussed in ASTM D21.06 technical committee meetings, representatives of the polish industry have indicated that extensive, long-term experimental data underpins the 0.5 criteria for the James Machine, but that due to potential liability, the industry is unable to produce it.

4.11.1.2 D3758

D3758, the *Standard Practice for Evaluation of Spray-Buff Products on Test Floors* (under the jurisdiction of technical committee D21 Polishes) was originally published in 1979. This document covers the comparison of spray-buff products (for use to maintain base floor-polish films) on test floors against a reference material. It specifies the use of a test method from the Chemical Specialties Manufacturers Association (CSMA) Bulletin Number 245–70 Comparative Determination Slip Resistance of Floor Polishes, now CSPA 0202 (see Chapter 5 — Other U.S. Standards and Guidelines).

This standard is under the jurisdiction of D21.04, the Performance Tests subcommittee.

4.11.2 D01 Paint and Related Coatings, Materials, and Applications

Established in 1902, D01 is responsible for over 670 standards, related to coating classification, sampling, preparation, application, analysis, quality assurance, and performance requirements.

4.11.2.1 D5859

D5859, the *Standard Test Method for Determining the Traction of Footwear on Painted Surfaces Using the VIT*, addresses a method of measuring the slip resistance of footwear (wet and dry) on painted walkway surfaces using the VIT. Although originally developed in D01, this document was subsequently transferred from D01 Paints to ASTM F13.10.

4.11.3 F15 Consumer Products

Formed in 1973, the purpose of F15 is to develop safety and performance standards for consumer products, a broad range of subjects including lighters, playground equipment, infant carriers, toys, beds, candles, scooters, and bathtubs. Recognizing that its work may overlap with that of other ASTM committees, the scope of F15 requires that it coordinate with committees having mutual interest in the subject of a given standard.

In the early 1970s, the need for slip resistance standards for bathtubs became apparent. As one of a number of products that had been identified as hazardous by the Consumer Product Safety Commission (CPSC), it was ranked 14th on the CPSC Product Hazard Index. ASTM formed Committee F15 Consumer Product Safety to develop such standards. Initial research conducted from 1973 to 1975 indicated that bathtubs far exceed shower stalls in terms of frequency and severity of injury. Most injuries were slips and falls entering or leaving the tub, or while changing between standing and sitting positions.

4.11.3.1 F462

F462 is the *Standard Consumer Safety Specification for Slip-Resistant Bathing Facilities* (under the jurisdiction of technical committee F15 Consumer Products).

At the time F462 was written, the only viable instruments available were the HPS, pendulum, James Machine, and the newly developed PAST (Brungraber Mark I or NBS-Brungraber). Through the process of elimination, primarily on practical grounds (i.e., insufficient space to operate an HPS, excessive speed of the pendulum, and inappropriate size/weight of the laboratory-based James Machine), the Brungraber Mark I was selected.

To establish a baseline and threshold for the test, 50 bathtub surfaces were tested, with individual results ranging from 0.003 to 0.417. As a result of this testing, the acceptable level of slip resistance was set as 0.04. The rationale was that the standard should be set at twice the value of the highest reading obtained on the untextured bathing surfaces tested.

The F462 standard calls for testing surfaces with the Brungraber Mark I PAST fitted with a Silastic 382 rubber test pad (medical grade), performed with soapy water (using Federal Specification P-S-624g or ASTM D799-74 specifications). Measurements are made in nine specific areas of the tub, and all nine areas must meet or exceed the threshold for the tub to pass. The bathtub meets the specification if slip resistance reads .04, bearing no known relationship to a threshold of safety for human ambulation.

Standard F462 was first approved in 1979, and has been reapproved several times (most recently in 1999). Reapproval means that, except for editorial changes, the standard was renewed without changes.

The primary problem is that the soap scum builds up on the tub surface due to soap and shampoo interaction with water hardness and other contaminants; this results in a smooth coating over the slip-resistant surface. The bather is not standing on the textured surface that was tested, but is standing on the soap scum film, which levels the texture significantly, reducing its slip resistance. Also, the consistency of the soapy water mixture is problematic. Even if a consistent product were easily available, the resulting mixture does not represent anything that occurs between a bather's foot and the tub surface while showering.

ASTM requires that any specification that includes a test method must contain all the requirements of a test method. The major portion of F462 is a detailed test method. The document has no precision and bias (P&B) statement. P&B is fundamental to validating a test method. Without it, there is no support that the protocol specified in the standard is any more accurate or appropriate than another.

4.11.4 C21 Ceramic Whitewares and Related Products

Established in 1948, C21 is responsible for more than 65 standards, primarily related to raw materials, physical and chemical testing, and performance and specifications relating to products of ceramic materials. Subcommittee C21.06 Ceramic Tile has jurisdiction over 15 standards involving such properties as bond strength, warpage, color, abrasion resistance, shock resistance, and electrical resistance.

4.11.4.1 C1028

C1028 is the *Standard Test Method for Determining the Static COF of Ceramic Tile and Other Like Surfaces by the Horizontal Dynamometer Pull-Meter Method* (under the jurisdiction of technical committee C21, Ceramic Tile) (see Figure 4.12).

Although it is often confused with the F609 HPS device (because it operates in a similar way), this is a different instrument. ASTM first published the document in 1984. A do-it-yourself instrument, the C1028 method consists of instructions on how to construct and operate the device, calling for an analog dynamometer, a Neolite test pad, plywood, and a 50-lb weight. Issues with the C1028 method include the following:

- Because it is not a manufactured device, almost every unit made is different from another, increasing the potential for variability of results.
- Although it is currently approved for wet testing, it has been long known that, similar to other dragsled technologies, the C1028 method produces erratic results on wet surfaces.
- As a manually operated instrument, it is more subject to operator influence than mechanically operated apparatus. Understandably, it is difficult to pull a 50-lb weight at a uniform speed without creating an erratic, jerking motion.
- C1028 cites a standard (HS-3) from the Rubber Manufacturers Association (RMA). According to the RMA, it no longer represents the footwear industry in any capacity; therefore, all standards, such as HS-3, have been withdrawn and are out of circulation.
- The Significance and Use section of C1028 states that the standard is for laboratory use and "should not be used to determine slip resistance under

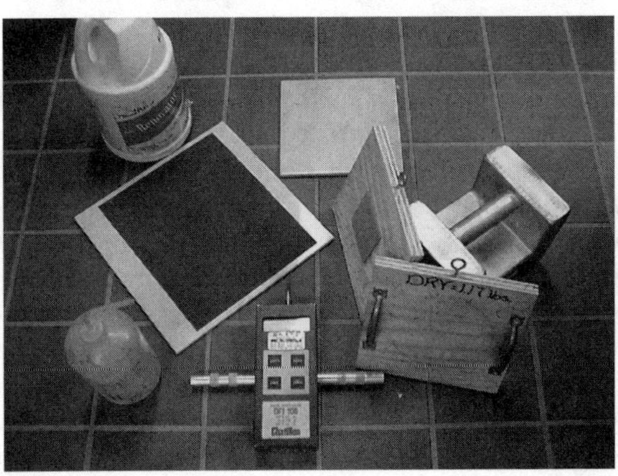

FIGURE 4.12 The materials needed to construct a horizontal pull dynamometer pull meter.

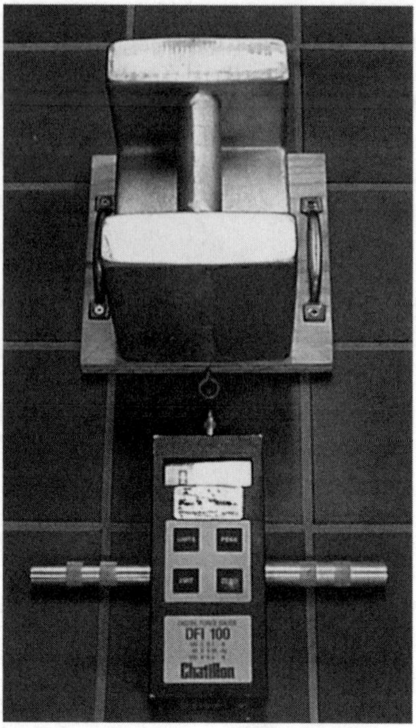

FIGURE 4.13 A C1028 apparatus fully assembled and ready to use.

field conditions." The rationale for this statement is that the test method was originally intended (similar to that of D2047) to establish the merchantability of new flooring-related products, not to assess the slip resistance of actual walkway surfaces (see Figure 4.13).

- The minimal detail provided for an instrument that must be constructed by the user can only lead to increased variability in design — and, therefore, results. The design of the apparatus should be as specific as possible to minimize variability in results. Design details that are not specified, but should be, include:
  - Type of wood and size/type of eyelet to be used (e.g., plywood, $^3/_4$-in. stainless steel eyelet)
  - Configuration of weight (e.g., dimensions can impact results)
  - Location of eyelet (e.g., dead center on a side of plywood base, with the grain)
  - Positioning of the Neolite pad on the bottom of the wood base (e.g., dead center) and method of attachment (e.g., epoxy, double-sided tape)
  - Positioning of the weight on the wood base (e.g., dead center, with narrow end facing toward the front)
- Method of securing the sandpaper when preparing Neolite and determining when the sandpaper should be replaced (e.g., when noticeably worn)
- A diagram showing dimensions and components should be provided as an appendix to the standard — This would help to ensure that all

instruments are constructed of the same materials in the same manner, thus reducing variability in results.

Despite these shortcomings and limitations, some vendors of flooring-related products that are supposed to be slip resistant often misuse this test method (see Slip Resistant Floor Treatment Study 2000, Exhibit 6.1).

As of 2002, work was under way by a task group of ASTM C21 to update this standard. Initial ballots of the revisions indicate that the committee is considering the removal of wet testing from the scope of the standard. It is also likely that the portion of the standard specifying the C1028 calibration tile will be eliminated because this tile is no longer available, and no replacement is available.

4.11.5 Summary

This array of standards has developed over time; it often disagrees and conflicts. Until recently, no single focal point of slip resistance standards existed, even within ASTM. So, the C21 Ceramic Tile task group was free to develop a standard that it felt the industry needed, and the D21 Polishes task group did the same. Over the course of many years, the committees closely guarded these standards, which permeated these respective industries. At the same time, as our knowledge and technology have progressed, the usefulness of these standards has diminished.

To streamline the process of standardization in this area, ASTM formally designated Technical Committee F13 as the only source for the development of slip resistance test methods. The rationale was that F13 was well positioned in terms of scope and expertise to develop "generic" test methods for slip resistance. Other committees with specialized needs (e.g., ceramic, resilient, polish, paint) could then reference the appropriate F13 standard and craft documents that included supplementary information (e.g., specimen preparation, thresholds, limits) for their application.

4.12 A WORK IN PROGRESS: THE ASTM "GOLD" STANDARD

Currently, there is no harmonization of pedestrian slip resistance test methods. The results of one tribometer cannot be correlated to the results of another. ASTM has undertaken an effort to resolve these differences by means of a proposed approach that is based on the relative ranking of materials against a reference set of materials.

Reference materials would consist of a single test foot material, under which a set of different test surfaces would be tested. Besides having different slip resistance values, falling within the range of the human perception of traction, the slip resistance values (and, therefore, the rank order) of the reference materials should remain constant, regardless of the apparatus.

At the site of the evaluation, each of reference surfaces would be tested and recorded, ensuring that they are ranked in the proper order. Next, the walkway surface in question would be tested with the same test foot used against the reference materials (see Figure 4.14).

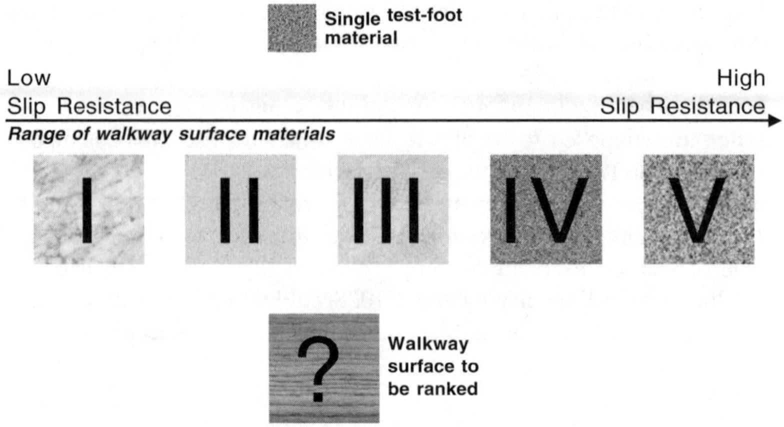

FIGURE 4.14 Primary ASTM "gold standard" methodology.

The walkway surface would be ranked against the set of reference materials. For example, assume that five reference materials are used, ranging in values between 0.18 and 0.73, and the results of the walkway surface in question is 0.35. That places the walkway surface of interest between two of the reference materials. The test results might be expressed by its relative ranking to the reference materials (e.g., 1 to 2), not the numerical results of the slipmeter.

Historically, a single friction coefficient was considered to differentiate between slip resistant and nonslip-resistant walkways. More recently, the slip resistance value is considered relative to the type of activities expected on the walkway surface. For example, dancers on a dance floor require *less* friction than do pedestrians, and workers pushing heavy loads across a floor require *more* friction. So, it is likely that no single threshold, such as the frequently cited 0.5 figure, is sufficient to appropriately distinguish slippery from tractive in all instances (see Figure 4.15).

This proposed test method, as a relative ranking against a uniform set of external calibration materials, has strong potential for standardization of slip resistance results at the international level for several reasons. The approach:

Tribometer Friction Test Results	Reference Material Pair
0.18	I
0.29	II
0.35	Test Result (II-III)
0.46	III
0.59	IV
0.73	V

FIGURE 4.15 ASTM "gold standard" ranking.

- Is not hardware dependent, thereby eliminating the need to develop multiple standards and permitting any tribometer, provided it can meet the performance criteria specified
- Standardizes a set of reference materials for testing.
- Eliminates the variety of scales used to report slip resistance results, thereby reducing confusion and misinterpretation

4.13 OTHER GROUNDBREAKING RESEARCH

Work under way at the Department of Biokinesiology and Physical Therapy at the University of Southern California (USC) (http://pt.usc.edu/labs/mbrl/) promises to settle longstanding debates regarding thresholds of slip resistance. With access to the latest equipment and the expertise to apply it effectively, the project, headed by Dr. Chris Powers, Director of the Musculoskeletal Biomechanics Research Laboratory at USC (and chair of ASTM F13 subcommittee F13.40 on research), is expected to relate slipmeter readings to human ambulation through a series of trials involving people walking across a set of force plates. This approach may also provide the basis for slip resistance bias (e.g., an accepted reference value).

Walking subjects cross a floor area several times at a normal gait while wearing goggles that do not permit the subject to see the floor. The subject is unaware of the location of the force plates or that a force plate was lubricated, thus resulting in a natural and unbiased slip. The walker is harnessed to an overhead trolley to prevent injury, but even this is set up to measure the degree of vertical support used in recovery from the slip. Features of this project that make it unique from other research include:

- Powerful computer modeling is used to study slip events.
- Subjects are unaware of floor conditions, thus providing realistic and unbiased results.
- Slipmeter readings are taken close to the subject's point of slip immediately following each event.
- Seven digital video cameras are set up to capture the motion of key portions of the subject's movements, using infrared markers located on the walking subject that allow for analysis from a variety of angles.

This is an ongoing project, and some portions of this work will probably be available for publication in 2003. For more information, see http://pt.usc.edu/labs/mbrl/research/slip.html.

EXHIBIT 4.1
COMPARISON CHART: U.S. RECOGNIZED SLIP RESISTANCE TEST METHODS

COMPARISON CHART: U.S. RECOGNIZED SLIP RESISTANCE TEST METHODS

Apparatus	Type	Yr	Avail	Wet	US Standard	P	Wt	L	Pad	OD	Cost	More Information
James	AS	40s	Y	N	ASTM F489 D2047 UL 410	N	N/A	M	Leather, Silastic	H	13-23,000	http://www.cspa.org (plans for manual apparatus) http://www.performnceadditives.com/jamztest.htm http://www.astm.org (Committees F13.10, D21.06)
HPS	DS	60s	Y	N	ANSI/ASTM F609 ANSI A1264.2	Y	10	W	Neolite	M	N/A	http://www.astm.org (Committee F13.10) http://www.trusty-step.com
PAST (Mark I)	AS	70s	N	N	ANSI/ASTM F1678 ASTM F462 ANSI 1264.2	Y	Unk	W	Leather	L	Unk	Slip Test, Inc. (Sliptestin@aol. com) http://www.astm.org (Committees F13.10, F15.03) Patent 3,975,940 – owned by the US
C1028	DS	80s	Y~	Y	ASTM C1028	Y	53	M	Neolite	H	300	http://www.astm.org (Committee C21.06)
PIAST (Mark II)	AS	80s	Y	Y	ANSI/ASTM F1677 NFPA 1901 ANSI A1264.2 OSHA 1926.754	Y	Unk	W	Neolite	L	4000	Slip Test, Inc. (Sliptestin@aol. com) http://www.astm.org (Committee F13.10) Patents 4,759,209 and 4,798,080
VIT (XL)	AS	90s	Y	Y	ASTM F1679, D5859 NFPA 1901 ANSI A1264.2 OSHA 1926.754	Y	4	W	Neolite	L	3200	http://www.englishxl.com http://www.astm.org (Committee F13.10) Patent 5,245,856

- Type: AS – Articulated Strut, DS – Dragsled, P – Pendulum
- Yr – decade in which the apparatus was developed
- Avail – Commercially Available
- Wet – Approved by US Standards for wet and dry testing
- P – Portable
- Wt – Approximate weight in pounds (field devices only)
- L – Listed for walkway surfaces or product merchantability
- OD – Operator Dependent (for velocity, force, angle – or complexity of set-up) – Low, Moderate, High
- Cost – Approximate Cost
- Unk – Unknown

NOTES
- ~ There is no manufacturer for this device. It must be constructed.
- ` (1) manual propelled, (2) electrically propelled, (3) Jablonsky enhancement, and (4) computerized version (Michelman)

EXHIBIT 4.2
COMPARISON CHART: SLIP RESISTANCE TEST METHODS NOT RECOGNIZED IN THE U.S.

COMPARISON CHART: SLIP RESISTANCE TEST METHODS NOT RECOGNIZED IN THE U.S.

Apparatus	A	Stnds	P	C	Pad	OD	Cost	More Information
DRAG SLED CLASS INSTRUMENTS								
PATENTED INSTRUMENTS								
Walker				US	Various	HP		Patent 2,225,140 (May, 1939)
Davies				US	Various	CR		Patent 3,187,552 (June, 1965)
Surface Friction Analyzer				US	Rubber	SP		Patent 3,828,605 (August, 1974), Fazekas – owned by Elias Productions
Majcherczyk	N	None	Y	Fr	Various	MD	N/A	Patent 4,4081,989 – owned by Centre Experimental de Recherches et d'Etudes du Batiment et des Travaux Publics
English UST				US	Neolite	MD		Prototype of a fully automated HPS, never commercially produced. Patent 4,8985,015 (January, 1990)
Pazzaglia				US	Various	HP		Patent 5,245,856 (September, 1993)
Welner				US	Various	MD		Patent 5,736,630 (April, 1998)
UNPATENTED INSTRUMENTS (MOTOR DRIVEN)								
Perma	Y	None	Y	US	Leather		Unk	http://www.perma.com
UFTM	N	None	Y	US	Various		N/A	Rotational movement of two 1" diameter test feet, developed by NIOSH in the 1970's – never commercially produced
Topaka	N	None	Y	US	Paper		N/A	see Chapter 5
Kett 94 Ai	Y	None	Y	Jap	Brass		3700	Japanese Patent http://www.kett.co.jp/e/products/pro6/94i.html, http://www.kett.com
In-tech Slip Meter	Y	None	Y	UK	Unknown		350	Allied Ltd – UK Patent applied for http://www.allied.dial.pipex.com/slipmeter.htm
Hoechst	N	None	N	Ger	Metal	MD	N/A	
Trusty Step HPS	Y	None	Y	US	Various		Unk	Similar to HPS (F609), http://www.trusty-step.com
Grip Meter	Y	None	Y	UK	Unk		Unk	http://www.anti-slip.com/
Tortus Etal	Y	AS/NZ	Y	UK	4S		3000	http://www.mastrad.com/ http://www.severnscience.co.uk/ — Overstates wet results. Includes Tortus II, FSC 2000, and Gabbrielli variations.
Sellmaier	Y	None	Y	Ger	Various		3500	Unreliable on wet surfaces, convex test pads, similar to Tortus devices Pioneer Eclipse Corporation
CEBTP Skidmeter	N	None	Y	Fr	Tire Rubber		N/A	A dragsled pull along two rails, controlled by a motor and gearbox

EXHIBIT 4.3
NEOLITE PATENT

COMPARISON CHART: SLIP RESISTANCE TEST METHODS NOT RECOGNIZED IN THE U.S.
(continued)

DRAG SLED CLASS INSTRUMENTS									
Apparatus	A	Stnds	P	C	Pad	OD	Cost	More Information	
UNPATENTED INSTRUMENTS (HAND OPERATED)									
ASM 725	Y	None	Y	US	Neolite	HP	800	http://www.americanslipmeter.com	Manually pulled devices result in undue operator influence
GMG 100	N	None	Y	Ger	Various	HP	N/A	http://www.hvbg.de/d/bia/starte.htm	
Static Friction Tester	N	None	Y	US	Unk	HP	N/A	Measurement Products Company (5 pound weight)	
Schuster	Y	Non-US	Y	Ger	Unk	HP	Unk	Unk	
Model 80	Y	None	Y	US	Leather	HP	1000	Technical Products Company	
PTI Drag Sled	N	None	Y	US	Various	HP	N/A	Pennsylvania Transportation Institute (PTI) Tester was used in trials for ADA – never commercial produced, Bohdan T. Kulakowski, Phd - Penn State btk1@psu.edu	

- Tortus Etal (incl varieties such as Gabbrielli, FSC 2000, Tortus II), UFTM – Universal Friction Testing Machine
- A – Commercially Available
- P – Portable
- C – Country of Origin
- OD – Operator Dependent (HP – hand pulled, CR – cranked, and SP – spring driven are more operator dependent than MD – motor driven
- Unk - Unknown

+ dragsled class instruments are subject to sticktion, and are invalid for wet testing

5 Other U.S. Standards and Guidelines

5.1 INTRODUCTION

Although the American Society for Testing and Materials (ASTM) is the most active in development of pedestrian safety related standards in the U.S., it is by no means the only one. Beyond the work of ASTM, a variety of federal government documents (e.g., Occupational Safety and Health Administration [OSHA], military, federal specifications) and other consensus standards (e.g., National Fire Protection Association [NFPA], American National Standards Institute [ANSI]) are available, in addition to work by private industry.

When referring to U.S.-developed regulations, standards, and specifications, it is important to understand several aspects of these documents: the perspective and biases of the developer, the stated and intended focus of the document (which oftentimes is quite narrow), and the method by which the document came to be (see Chapter 8, Exhibit 8.2 "Summary of Organizations Developing Standards in the Field of Slip Resistance").

5.2 OCCUPATIONAL SAFETY AND HEALTH ADMINISTRATION (OSHA)

OSHA refers to three separate slip resistance standards, each promulgated at different times and with varying degrees of enforceability. This information can be reviewed at the OSHA Web site http://www.osha.gov.

5.2.1 Section 1910.22 General Requirements

Recommendation: Federal Register, April 1, 1990, Vol. 55, No. 69, p. 13408, 29 CFR, *Walking and Working Surfaces and Personal Protective Equipment (Fall Protection Systems); Notice of Proposed Rulemaking — Section 1910.22 General Requirements (Appendix A to Subpart D Compliance Guidelines)*

1. Surface conditions.

2. Slip-resistance. A reasonable measure of slip-resistance is static coefficient of friction (COF). A COF of 0.5, which is based upon studies by the University of Michigan and reported in "Work Surface Friction Definitions, Laboratory and Field Measurements, and a Comprehensive Bibliography," is recommended as a guide to achieve proper slip resistance. A COF of 0.5 is not intended to be an absolute standard value. A higher

COF may be necessary for certain work tasks, such as carrying objects, pushing or pulling objects, or walking up or down ramps.

Slip-resistance can vary from surface to surface, or even on the same surface, depending upon surface conditions and employee footwear. Slip-resistant flooring material such as textured, serrated, or punched surfaces and steel grating may offer additional slip-resistance. These types of floor surfaces should be installed in work areas that are generally slippery because of wet, oily, or dirty operations. Slip-resistant type footwear may also be useful in reducing slipping hazards.

The OSHA 1910 "standard" for slip resistance is not a law, nor is it a standard. It is a proposed nonmandatory appendix item that has yet to be adopted as a standard (it specifies a slip resistance of 0.50 or higher for the workplace). Although it is possible for an OSHA inspector to cite this guideline under the "General Duty Clause," this is a rare occurrence. What makes this particularly difficult is that OSHA has not specified a test protocol or device upon which to base a citation, effectively making it of questionable enforceability.

5.2.2 Manlifts 1910.68(c)(3)(v)

Surfaces. The upper or working surfaces of the step shall be of a material having inherent nonslip characteristics (coefficient of friction not less than 0.5) or shall be covered completely by a nonslip tread securely fastened to it.

Again, this reference specifies no test protocol or device as a basis for a citation, and thus is an arguably unenforceable regulation (see http://www.osha-slc.gov/OshStd_data/1910_0068.html).

5.2.3 1926 Subpart R — Steel Erection Regulatory (3)

Slip resistance of skeletal structural steel. Workers shall not be permitted to walk the top surface of any structural steel member installed after (5 years after effective date of final rule) that has been coated with paint or similar material unless documentation or certification that the coating has achieved a minimum average slip resistance of 0.50 when measured with an English XL tribometer or equivalent tester on a wetted surface at a testing laboratory is provided. Such documentation or certification shall be based on the appropriate ASTM standard test method conducted by a laboratory capable of ASTM standard test method conducted by a laboratory capable of performing the test. The results shall be available at the site and to the steel erector. (Appendix B to this subpart references appropriate ASTM standard test methods that may be used to comply with this paragraph (c)(3)).

Appendix B to Subpart R – Acceptable Test Methods for Testing Slip-Resistance of Walking/Working Surfaces (1926.754(c)(3)). Non-Mandatory Guidelines for Complying with 1926.754(c)(3).

The following references provide acceptable test methods for complying with the requirements of 1926.754(c)(3).

- *Standard Test Method for Using a Portable Inclineable Articulated Strut Tester (PIAST)(ASTM F1677–96).*

- *Standard Test Method for Using a Variable Incidence Tribometer (VIT)(ASTM F1679–96).*

OSHA announced that the final Steel Erection Standard was to go into effect on January 18, 2002. Although implementation is not required for 5 years from this date, this standard specifes a threshold and acceptable test methods with which to establish compliance. For a more thorough discussion on the rationale and science that resulted in these specifications, see the OSHA Structural Steel Standard Commentary in Exhibit 5.1. As of this writing, all states except three, which administer their own job safety programs, have put the steel erection standard (or a more stringent version) into effect.

5.3 AMERICANS WITH DISABILITIES ACT (ADA)

Public Law 101–336, 7/26/90. Federal Register Vol. 56, No. 144, Chapter A4.5.1, Friday, July 26, 1991 Rules & Regulations (http://www.usdoj.gov/crt/ada/adahom1.htm)

The ADA provisions for slip resistance, like OSHA, were also developed as a guideline, since the specification appears in an appendix. Because no test protocol, apparatus, or test foot material is specified, it is difficult to apply them. The ADA specifies slip resistance of at least 0.60 for level surfaces and 0.80 for ramps, where accessible by persons with disabilities.

These thresholds were established based on a flawed two-phase research sponsored by the Architectural and Transportation Barriers Compliance Board (ATBCB). The first phase of the study involved five able-bodied individuals walking at fast speeds in dissimilar footwear over a clean, dry force plate and the use of a "detergent-wetted" NBS-Brungraber (PAST, or Mark I) with a Silastic 382 rubber test pad (similar to ASTM F462 for bathtub evaluation). In another phase of the study, nine mobility-disabled subjects walked across a force plate. Because this study was of such a limited scope, it was inappropriate to arrive at any thresholds for the general population (Fendley and Marpet, 1996).

According to correspondence dated January 19, 1993 from the Assistant Attorney General John R. Dunne:

> *There are no enforceable standards for coefficients of friction in the regulations. The Appendix to the Guidelines, which is advisory only, discusses recommended coefficients of friction in section A4.5.1 (page 35,678) . . . the recommended coefficients of friction are provided only as advisory guidance and not as regulatory requirements.*

On November 16, 1999, the slip resistance specifications of 0.6 and 0.8 were removed. As of this writing, revised criteria are still pending.

5.3.1 A4.5 GROUND AND FLOOR SURFACES/A4.5.1 GENERAL

People who have difficulty walking or maintaining balance or who use crutches, canes, or walkers, as well as those with restricted gaits are particularly sensitive to slipping and tripping hazards. For such people, a stable and regular surface is necessary for safe walking, particularly on stairs. Wheelchairs can be propelled most easily on surfaces that are hard, stable, and regular. Soft, loose surfaces such as shag carpet, loose sand or gravel, wet clay, and irregular surfaces such as cobblestones can significantly impede wheelchair movement.

Slip resistance is based on the frictional force necessary to keep a shoe heel or crutch tip from slipping on a walking surface under conditions likely to be found on the surface. Whereas the dynamic coefficient of friction during walking varies in a complex and nonuniform way, the static COF, which can be measured in several ways, provides a close approximation of the slip resistance of a surface. Contrary to popular belief, some slippage is necessary to walking, especially for persons with restricted gaits; a truly "non-slip" surface could not be negotiated.

OSHA recommends that walking surfaces have a static COF of 0.5. A research project sponsored by the ATBCB (Access Board) conducted tests with persons with disabilities and concluded that a higher COF was needed by such persons. A static COF of 0.6 is recommended for accessible routes and 0.8 for ramps.

It is recognized that the COF varies considerably due to the presence of contaminants, water, floor finishes, and other factors not under the control of the designer or builder and not subject to design and construction guidelines and that compliance would be difficult to measure on the building site. Nevertheless, many common building materials suitable for flooring are now labeled with information on the static COF. Although it may not be possible to compare one product directly with another, or to guarantee a constant measure, builders and designers are encouraged to specify materials with appropriate values. As more products include information on slip resistance, improved uniformity in measurement and specification is likely. The Access Board's advisory guidelines on Slip Resistant Surfaces provide additional information on this subject.

5.4 ACCESS BOARD RECOMMENDATIONS

The ATBCB (or Access Board) (http://www.access-board.gov/publications/4-SlipResistantSurfaces/A9.html) of the U.S. Department of Justice was created to ensure federal agency compliance with the Architectural Barriers Act (ABA). The Access Board adopted the ADA recommendations, and has stated these specifications as a guideline, not a requirement or a standard. Again, no test protocol (e.g., device or test method) is specified.

5.5 FEDERAL SPECIFICATIONS

5.5.1 RR-G-1602D

RR-G-1602D is the Federal Specification for *Grating, Metal, Other than Bar Type (Floor, Except for Naval Vessels)*. Originally published in 1970 (current version dated 1996), this specification is a procedure for testing the slip resistant characteristics of metal gratings used in floor surfaces within military and General Services Administration (GSA) applications. Threshold values range from approximately 0.34 to 0.49 depending on the material (e.g., aluminum, steel), condition (dry, mud, ice, grease, detergent), and test foot material (leather, boot rubber, shoe rubber, Neolite®, and Hypolon) where such flooring is subject to foot traffic. The test method specified is a homemade equivalent to a C1028 instrument, using a 3-in. diameter sole material, a dead weight of 175 lbs, and a "continuous recorder to record the resistance offered by the grating to the material." Section 3.7 provides thresholds of "anti-slip," and Section 4.4.3 specifies the test materials and method.

5.6 U.S. MILITARY SPECIFICATIONS (NAVY)

The following specifications prescribe the use of a horizontal slip tester.

5.6.1 MIL-D-23003A(SH)

This military specification refers to *Deck Covering Compound, Nonslip, Rollable.*

5.6.2 MIL-D-24483A

This military specification refers to *Nonslip Flight Deck Compound.*

5.6.3 MIL-D-0016680C (Ships) and MIL-D-18873B

These military specifications are for Deck Covering Magnesia Aggregate Mixture. These specifications both provide static coefficient of friction (SCOF) and dynamic coefficient of friction (DCOF) thresholds of 0.3 to 0.6 (against dry leather and rubber, respectively) and 0.4 to 0.6 (against wet leather and rubber). They specify the use of either generic inclined plane or dragsled-type instruments.

5.6.4 MIL-D-3134J

This military specification for *Deck Covering Materials (1988),* outlines procedures for testing under dry, wet (with 4% salt), and oily (SAE 10W) conditions using leather and rubber test pads. Although the test method options are the same as 18873B (see Section 5.6.3), the thresholds vary.

5.6.5 MIL-D-17951C (Ships)

A 1975 specification, this military specification for *Deck Covering, Lightweight, Nonslip, Silicon Carbide Particle Coated Fabric, Film, or Composite, and Sealing Compound supercedes*the 1961 version. Thresholds are similar to those of 18873B (see Section 5.6.3).

5.6.6 MIL-W-5044C

A 1970 specification, this military specification for *Walkway Compound, Nonslip, and Walkway Matting, Nonslip* supercedes the 1964 version. Describing a homemade dragsled device, it specifies a variety of thresholds, depending on the type of surface, the condition (dry, water, oil), and the type of slider (leather, rubber). Thresholds range from 0.45 to 1.00.

5.7 NFPA INTERNATIONAL (FORMERLY NATIONAL FIRE PROTECTION ASSOCIATION)

NFPA is a nonprofit organization founded in 1896 http://www.nfpa.org. With more than 75,000 members, NFPA's mission is to reduce fire and other hazards by developing and advocating scientifically based consensus codes and standards. NFPA maintains more than 300 consensus codes and standards in 250 technical committees with more than 6000 members, many of which are used as a basis for legislation and regulation nationally and internationally.

NFPA operates on a full consensus basis, meaning that committee balance (preventing one interest from dictating the committee's agenda), transparency (public review of draft documents), and consensus are required elements in the process.

5.7.1 NFPA 1901

NFPA 1901 is the *Standard for Automotive Fire Apparatus*. This standard (Section 13-7.3) recognizes the use of the variable incidence tribometer (VIT, or English XL™) for all surfaces used for stepping, standing, or walking on new mobile fire apparatus. It establishes a minimum average slip resistance as follows:

- 0.68 for *exterior surfaces (wet)* when measured per ASTM F1679 (English XL VIT). It was subsequently amended to also permit the use of the portable inclinable articulated strut slip tester (PIAST, or Brungraber Mark II), with thresholds of 0.52 (wet) when measured per ASTM F1677.
- 0.58 for *interior surfaces (dry)* when measured per ASTM F1679 and 0.47 (dry) when measured per ASTM F1677.

5.7.2 NFPA 101/5000

Updated every 3 years, the 2003 edition of NFPA 101 (and 5000, NFPA's building code) is as vague as the other building codes with regard to slip resistance. However, the appendices of each of these documents (101-A7.1.6.4 and 500-A12–1.6.4) indicate that ASTM F1679 (VIT) and ASTM F1677 (PIAST) are acceptable methods for measuring the slip resistance of walkway surfaces and stair treads.

These standards specify that walkway surfaces are to be slip resistant under "foreseeable conditions." These appendices also make it clear that "foreseeable conditions" are those likely to be present in that area. The example is that a foreseeable condition of a swimming pool deck/area is that it will be wet.

5.8 AMERICAN NATIONAL STANDARDS INSTITUTE (ANSI)

Based in Washington, D.C., ANSI (http://www.ansi.org) has been the administrator and coordinator of U.S. voluntary standards for more than 80 years. It is a nonprofit organization. ANSI does not actually develop standards. Instead, it facilitates development by establishing consensus among qualified groups. More than 175 entities are accredited by ANSI to develop consensus standards. ANSI conducts scheduled audits to assure the standards process is being observed by accredited organizations. Currently, ANSI includes more than 1000 members. ANSI has also developed more than 16,000 standards.

ANSI is a founding member of and the official U.S. representative to the International Organization for Standardization (ISO) (see Chapter 7). ANSI participates in 78% of all ISO technical committees and is responsible for accrediting U.S. Technical Advisory Groups (U.S. TAGs), which develop and communicate U.S. positions on activities and ballots of the international technical committee. ANSI is also a member of the Pan American Standards Commission (COPANT).

ANSI standards are to be withdrawn if not revised or reaffirmed within 5 years (unless an extension has been granted). ANSI standards not revised or reaffirmed within 10 years are automatically withdrawn.

5.8.1 A1264.2-2001

A1264.2-2001 is the *Standard for the Provision of Slip Resistance on Walking/Working Surfaces*.

The American Society of Safety Engineers (ASSE) acts as secretariat for this ANSI standard, which was officially adopted in August 2001. It differs from other slip resistance standards (such as those from ASTM International and Underwriters Laboratories) in that it is oriented to workplaces instead of public places, and it specifies a numeric threshold of safety for walking. It is the only standard aside from the James Machine standard for polished surfaces (ASTM D2047) to set a minimum value.

The goal of the standard is to provide criteria to businesses in order to reduce the potential for employee slips and falls. Although it can be considered a state-of-the-art standard, revisions to this standard will be necessary as advances in the field are made. The standard provides for the minimum performance requirements necessary for increased safety on walking/working surfaces in the workplace. Because many workplaces are also subject to pedestrian foot traffic from the public, the standard can also deliver similar benefits in reducing the potential for public liability.

In some instances, the standard refers the user to other ANSI and ASTM documents for further details. Due to the broad scope and many specifications provided or referenced in A1264.2, support from a knowledgeable and experienced safety consultant can provide constructive and valuable assistance. Three basic areas are addressed by the standard: provisions for reducing hazards, test procedures and equipment, and a slip resistance guideline.

Provisions for Reducing Hazards

- Footwear applications and considerations for the work environment, including traction
- Location, design, and maintenance of mats and runners, including special considerations for high hazard areas
- Housekeeping and maintenance procedures, including requirements of training, staff supervision, and floor monitoring

- Pre- and postincident warnings, including signage/symbols, and placement
- Controlled access, including barricades and containing hazards
- Selection of walkway surface materials, including discussion of floor finishing and treatment options
- Snow and ice control and removal

Test Procedures and Equipment

- ASTM International test methods
- Dry surfaces equipment
- Test equipment for wet or contaminated surfaces

Slip Resistance Guideline (Dry)

- Acceptable test methods
- Test foot material specifications
- A threshold of safety guideline for dry walkway surfaces of 0.5

5.8.2 A137.1-1988

This ANSI standard, *Specifications for Ceramic Tile,* references ASTM C1028 as the method for determining slip resistance qualities of ceramic tile.

5.9 UNDERWRITERS LABORATORIES

Established in 1894, Underwriters Laboratories Inc. (UL) is an independent, nonprofit product safety testing and certification organization (see http://www.ul.com and http://ulstandardsinfonet.ul.com [standards search]). UL maintains more than 750 standards.

Until recently, the UL standards process was a closed one. Only those specifically selected and invited to participate were involved. In an effort to be recognized as a true consensus standards-making organization, UL has recently elected to adopt ANSI standards development procedures.

UL now forms Standards Technical Panels (STPs), consisting of knowledgeable and interested parties with open meetings and drafts made available for public comment prior to publishing. Essentially, standards are developed by UL using the ANSI canvass method instead of the more comprehensive full-consensus method (see Chapter 8, Exhibit 8.2 Approaches to Development of Standards). UL is the largest ANSI accredited standards developer using the canvass method. As a result of using this new approach, UL documents are eligible for ANSI approval. Presently, the UL method of consensus does not appear to afford complete transparency, or a suitable means of universal public comment because documents proposed for approval must be purchased from UL in order to be reviewed.

5.9.1 UL 410

UL 410 is the standard for *Slip Resistance of Floor Surface Materials (as measured by the James Machine).*

Many products claim to be classified or certified by UL for slip resistance. Although UL does not "certify" products with respect to slip resistance, it does "classify" products as such. Around 1970, UL began the "classification" of some products instead of "listing" them as a way for UL to increase revenue through fees.

UL will apply the treatment to a surface and test it to UL 410, using the James Machine. To be permitted to use the UL Classification Marking, test results must meet or exceed the specified slip resistance threshold, and the manufacturer must pay a fee. In 1953, UL stopped releasing actual test results to applicants and now issues documentation only as to whether or not the results have exceeded the threshold. The average slip resistance threshold is set at a minimum of 0.5 for these products. The slip resistance for an individual surface is set at a minimum of 0.45.

A Classification Mark appears on products that UL has evaluated for specific properties, a limited range of hazards, or suitability for use under limited or special conditions. In the case of slip resistance, the product will display this notice:

> **CLASSIFIED BY UNDERWRITERS LABORATORIES INC.® AS TO SLIP RESISTANCE ONLY.**

This is a product standard that applies to the following types of floor surfaces and treatments:

- Floor covering materials made of wood or composite materials
- Water-based floor treatment materials
- Fillers, sealers, varnishes, and similar floor treatment materials
- Detergent materials
- Abrasive-grit-bearing floor treatment materials
- Floor treatment materials other than water-base
- Sweeping compound materials
- Walkway construction materials used as floor plates, ramps, and stair treads that are made of natural stone, composite materials, abrasive-grit surface materials, and metal

Thus, the scope of UL 410 is significantly broader than ASTM D2047, in that it is intended for use for virtually all types of walkway surfaces and finishes. It is important to understand that the intent of this standard was to provide for consistent laboratory testing under ideal conditions. According to James himself, the instrument was designed as a comparative method, to compare the results of a treated surface material to that of the same material untreated. While James did discuss the 0.5 threshold, it did not appear to be his intention to use his instrument and this threshold as a means to categorically differentiate a slip resistant surface from a non-slip-resistant surface.

In its current form, UL 410 has numerous drawbacks that impede its viability as a valid test method (also see Chapter 4, Section 4.4 and Section 4.11.1.1):

- No provisions are recommended for calibration of the instrument. This is an essential step for the manually propelled version of the instrument, the only (and most operator-dependent) version covered under this document.
- The document permits wet and contaminated testing, although the literature repeatedly demonstrates that the apparatus is subject to sticktion.

- Unlike ASTM, UL documents require no testing to validate the protocol or apparatus. Thus, there is no precision and bias statement (P&B) (nor, to date, has one been planned) to support the accuracy or repeatability of the test method.
- The document calls for the use of leather, a highly variable substance inappropriate for wet or contaminated testing. UL 410 does not even specify standard leather (government specification KK-L-165), allowing the introduction of yet another unaccounted-for variable.
- With one exception, the substrates (or floor materials on which floor treatments are tested) are not standardized, adding still another variable.

The following limitations must also be kept in mind when considering a UL classification as to slip resistance:

- The James Machine is a laboratory device designed to test under ideal conditions only for the suitability of new flooring products. This standard is not approved for field testing. There is no guarantee that the results of the installed material will be the same as those in the laboratory.
- Most important, the James Machine was not designed for wet testing or for materials other than smooth, untextured surfaces.
- Calculations in the design do not account for the added weight of the substantial struts, thereby introducing an uncorrected variable.
- Given that the substrate (the tile used to test the treatment) is often 0.5 to start within its untreated condition, the treatment need only be neutral and does not have to degrade the slip resistance in order to pass.

5.10 MODEL BUILDING CODES

Primary specifications relating to slip resistance and dimensional criteria for pedestrian safety are contained in *Section 10 — Means of Egress* (also see Chapter 1). Whereas each of these codes requires that walkway surfaces and stair treads be slip resistant, none provide requirements or even guidance on acceptable thresholds or methods of assessing slip resistance.

5.11 OBSOLETE STANDARDS

5.11.1 Federal Test Method Standard 501a, Method 7121

This is the standard for *Floor Covering, Resilient, Non-Textile; Sample and Testing*.

First published in June 1966 and withdrawn many years ago, this government test method specified the Sigler pendulum device to measure dynamic COF for nearly 20 years. The scope of the document was the measurement of DCOF for resilient non-textile floor coverings with relatively smooth surfaces using rubber (Standard Reference Compound No. 3 in method 14111 of Federal Test Method

Standard No. 601, for rubber test heel and leather [Federal Specification KK-L-165]) (http://www.fss.gsa.gov/pub/fedspecs/sort2.cfm).

5.11.2 U.S. General Services Administration Specification P-F-430C(1)

This is the *Finish, Floor, Water Emulsion standard.*

This government specification, in place for many years, required that floor finishes meet a 0.5 static COF requirement using the James Machine. It was canceled in July 1999 (http://www.fss.gsa.gov/pub/fedspecs/sort5c.cfm).

5.11.3 ASTM D4518-91

ASTM D4518-91 is the *Standard Test Method for Measuring Static Friction of Coating Surfaces.* This standard was under the jurisdiction of D01 Paints. Originally published in 1985, this standard has since been withdrawn. It covered two separate methods: an Inclined Plane Test and the Horizontal Pull Test.

5.11.4 ASTM D-21 Gray Pages

In the early 1980s, ASTM Technical Committee D21 was unable to pass several test methods for alternatives to the James Machine. The methods were subsequently published in the gray pages of the Book of Standards (V 15.04):

- *Proposal P 125 Test Method for Static and Dynamic Coefficient of Friction of Polish-Coated Floor Surfaces as Measured by the Horizontal Slip Tester* (see ASTM F609)
- *Proposal P 126 Test Method for Static Coefficient of Friction of Polish-Coated Floor Surfaces as Measured by the NBS-Brungraber Articulated Arm Tester* (see ASTM F1678)
- *Proposal P 127 Test Method for Dynamic Coefficient of Friction of Polish-Coated Floor Surfaces as Measured by the NBS-Sigler Pendulum Impact Tester* (see Chapter 8 for more information on this apparatus)
- *Proposal P 128 Test Method for Static Coefficient of Friction of Polish-Coated Floor Surfaces as Measured by the Topaka Slip Tester* — A dragsled class of tribometer, this apparatus uses a 110-volt motor to pull a 5 in. × 8 in. canvas bag containing five pounds of lead shot across a walkway surface at 3.3 in. per second. Bond paper (25% rag content) is specified as test foot material instead of a footwear-bottom-related material. Similar to the HPS (F609), the weight is connected to the motor by a nylon cord and is fitted with three ½-inch diameter "rubber buttons" that contact the paper. No standard exists in the U.S. or abroad, although the instrument is now reportedly sold by a vendor of floor finish systems and is promoted as a valid test method.

5.12 U.S.-BASED INDUSTRY ASSOCIATIONS INVOLVED WITH SLIP RESISTANCE

5.12.1 Ceramic Tile Institute of America (CTIOA)

Some tile manufacturers and slip-resistant floor treatment vendors refer to meeting or exceeding requirements as required by the Ceramic Tile Institute (CTI) (http://www.thetiledoctor.com), an industry group representing the interests of the ceramic tile industry. Three primary goals in the CTIOA mission statement are:

- To promote appropriate and expanded use of ceramic tile and natural stone
- Develop and conduct educational, informational, and promotional programs
- Develop and disseminate technical and promotional publications (media)

Historically, CTIOA has specified the use of ASTM C1028, which is a test method only and does not specify a level of safety. C1028 cannot be exceeded, since it specifies no "safe" or "unsafe" level of slip resistance. However, CTIOA then adopted the James Machine guideline of.50, even though no known correlation exists between these instruments.

Recently, CTIOA released a series of position papers endorsing the use of non-U.S. slip resistance test methods: the ramp, the Tortus, and the pendulum (see Chapter 8), in place of the C1028. CTIOA endorses the thresholds listed in Table 5.1.

No thresholds are indicated for inclined surfaces (e.g., ramps).

Although no published peer-reviewed research is cited, the CTIOA primarily references a draft ISO standard (10545-17), a series of personal communications, and its own prior paper to support this position.

5.12.2 Consumer Specialty Products Association (CSPA)

Formerly the Chemical Specialty Manufacturers Association (CSMA) (http://www.cspa.org), the Consumer Specialty Products Association (CSPA) is the industry trade group representing the makers of formulated products for home and commercial use. It was formed in 1914. CSPA members total more than 220, and include companies engaged in the manufacture, formulation, distribution, and sale of consumer specialty products for household, institutional, and industrial use. CSPA member companies account for more than $14 billion in annual revenues.

TABLE 5.1
CTIOA Endorsed Slip Resistance Thresholds

Instrument	Test Foot	Condition	Locations	Threshold
Tortus	4S rubber	Wet	Level floors	0.50
			Bathtubs, showers, pool decks	0.70
Pendulum	4S rubber	Wet	Level floors	35 BPN
	TRRL rubber		Showers, pool decks	

One of CSPA's seven divisions is Polishes and Floor Maintenance, which performs research in the field of slip resistance. ASTM D3758, *Standard Practice for Evaluation of Spray-Buff Products on Test Floors,* refers to CSMA Bulletin Number 245–70 (Tentative Method), Comparative Determination Slip Resistance of Floor Polishes. This test method, established in 1970, is a subjective relative ranking of slip resistance, comparing coatings to another of accepted value. The test calls for a test subject to slide a clean sheet of writing paper across the floor with a shod foot, and rate the surfaces from 1 (little slip resistance) to 5 (high slip resistance). As of 2002, this test method was redesignated as CSPA 0202. The bulletin also states that CSMA considers any floor polish, tested by ASTM D2047, that also has a static COF of at least 0.5 to meet the requirements of the proposed FTC Rule 5; this would make it permissible to promote the product as "slip resistant" (see Chapter 3).

It is important to remember that this test method was not developed by a consensus of a balance of interested parties, but by an industry trade group with a mission to promote its members' products. CSPA is also a supplier (in some cases the only known supplier) of:

- Official vinyl composition tile (OVCT), required as a calibration surface for testing under ASTM D2047, and now available under the name TM-1, Vinyl Composition Tiles for Wax Testing
- Leather conforming to Federal Specification KK-L-665C, also required for the ASTM D2047 test method
- James Machine charts, a basic requirement for testing under any standard using this apparatus

CSPA is currently working on a code of conduct for the marketing of slip resistant floor treatments. The code of conduct is an attempt to keep manufacturers from making claims beyond what is technically possible with treatments and coatings of a slip resistant nature.

5.12.3 Resilient Floor Covering Institute (RFCI)

A coalition of seven of the largest manufacturers of resilient flooring, RFCI is an industry trade association of North American manufacturers (http://www.rfci.com). RFCI was established to support the interests of the resilient floor covering industry. Institute objectives include:

- Promoting the use of resilient floor covering as a product category
- Monitoring and responding to federal, state, and local legislation as well as regulations that affect the industry and its products

Most standards-making activities that interest RFCI are under the jurisdiction of ASTM Technical Committee F06, Resilient Floor Coverings; however, the issue of slip resistance test methods developed in ASTM F13 are also considered important enough to prompt RFCI's involvement. RFCI has conducted research regarding slip resistance test methods, but their work is not made public. As with other similar organizations, it must be understood that work done by RFCI is not performed by a balance of interested parties, but by an industry trade group with a mission to promote its members' products.

5.12.4 Footwear Industries of America (FIA)

Footwear Industries of America's (FIA) (now part of American Apparel and Footwear Association [AAFA]) (http://www.americanapparel.org) mission is realized through programs that help members maximize productivity, enhance marketing effectiveness, and ensure their voice in politics. It is the only national association for footwear manufacturers, importers and distributors, and suppliers to the leather and allied trades.

The purpose of the FIA Slip Resistant Footwear Committee is to study and evaluate the slip resistant qualities of footwear soling materials by testing with the four most recognized testing machines under varied conditions and surfaces. Task force groups are studying the following segments of slip resistance:

- Outsole compound and design
- Environment and conditions
- Testing methods
- Statistical analysis and data research

Members of FIA automatically become members of the world's largest footwear research and development organization, the SATRA Footwear Technology Centre, based in Kettering, England. SATRA has a contractual arrangement with FIA to provide technical information and products and services (see Section 8.10.2).

5.12.5 Contact Group on Slips, Trips, and Falls (CGSTF)

The CGSTF (http://www.safeworkresearch.com/slip/) is intended to provide an open forum for discussion on scientific matters related to slips, trips, and falls accidents. It will hopefully encourage direct exchange of experience between the participants; strengthen collaboration in the field of slip and fall research, training, and standardization; and help identify recent publications.

5.12.6 National Safety Council (NSC)

NSC (http://www.nsc.org) was founded in 1913 and chartered by Congress in 1953. Its mission is "to educate and influence society to adopt safety, health and environmental policies, practices and procedures that prevent and mitigate human suffering and economic losses arising from preventable causes." The Council is a nonprofit, nongovernmental, international public service organization dedicated to improving the safety, health, and environmental well-being of all people. As a nongovernment organization, the NSC does not have the authority to legislate or regulate.

The boards and their officers and committees, aided by some 2000 more volunteers, determine policies, operating procedures, and programs to be developed and carried out by the Council's professional staff of more than 300. Board members represent business, labor, Council Chapters, government, community groups, trade and professional associations, schools, and individuals. The Council's 37,000-member facilities employ more than 20 million people.

The NSC maintains more than 20 publications, programs, posters, and other materials related to slip and fall prevention, most of which consist of basic information.

5.12.7 American Academy of Forensic Sciences (AAFS)

With more than 5000 members, the AAFS (http://www.aafs.org/) consists of ten sections representing a wide range of forensic specialties. The Engineering Sciences Section deals with ergonomic and human biomechanical related issues, including slips and falls.

The AAFS publishes the *Journal of Forensic Sciences,* an internationally recognized scientific journal. AAFS also offers newsletters, an annual scientific meeting, and seminars. AAFS holds its annual scientific meeting in February, at which time more than 500 scientific papers, seminars, workshops, and other special events are presented. Professionals gather to present the most current information, research, and updates in this expanding field.

Through its journal and the annual meeting (which normally has a track of sessions devoted to slips and falls), AAFS has been the forum for many peer-reviewed research projects related to slip resistance and fall prevention.

EXHIBIT 5.1
OSHA REPORT ON SLIP RESISTANCE FOR STRUCTURAL STEEL

5214 Federal Register/Vol. 66, No. 12/Thursday, January 18, 2001/Rules and Regulations (pp. 5214–5218)

Paragraph (c)(3) will reduce the risk of steel erection workers slipping on coated steel members installed three years after the effective date of this standard. At that time, it will prohibit employees from walking on the top surface of any structural steel member that has been coated with paint or similar material, unless the coating has achieved a minimum average slip resistance of 0.50 when wet on an English XL tribometer, or the equivalent measurement on another device. This paragraph does not require that the particular coated member be tested. Rather, it requires the test to be done on a sample of the paint formulation produced by the paint manufacturer. The testing laboratory must use an acceptable ASTM method and an English XL tribometer or equivalent tester must be used on a wetted surface and the laboratory must be capable of employing this method. The test results must be available at the site and to the steel erector. Appendix B lists two appropriate ASTM standard test methods that may be used to comply with the paragraph. If other ASTM methods are approved, they too are allowed under this provision.

The final paragraph differs from the proposal in two significant respects. Proposed paragraph (c)(3) would have prohibited employees from walking on the top surface of any structural steel member with a finish coat that decreased the coefficient of friction (CoF) from that of the uncoated steel.

The final text sets a specific slip resistance for the coated surface, when tested wet. In addition, proposed paragraph (c)(3) stated that the paragraph applied to coated steel installed at the effective date of the standard, rather than, as in the final, three years later.

The Hazard

Based on SENRAC's discussions, and the rulemaking record, OSHA finds that working on steel surfaces coated with paint or other protective coatings presents slip and fall hazards to employees and that this standard must reduce this hazard using feasible means. SENRAC described the hazards as the use of paint or coatings on steel for structures exposed to highly corrosive materials (such as those used in mills and chemical plants) or exposed to varying weather conditions (such as stadiums). In the proposal, OSHA set out SENRAC's concerns as follows:

The Committee found that a major cause of falls in the steel erection industry is the presence of slippery walking, working and climbing surfaces in steel erection operations when fall protection is not used. The problem initially arises from the application of protective coatings on structural steel used, for example in the construction of mills, chemical plants and other structures exposed to highly corrosive materials as well as in the construction of stadiums or other structures exposed to varying weather conditions. It is usually impractical to leave the steel uncoated and then to paint the entire structure in the field after erection. Unfortunately, steel coated with paints or protective coatings can be extremely slippery. When there is moisture, snow, or ice on coated steel, the hazard is increased ... (63 FR 43467).

As discussed below regarding/1926.760, accident data in this record demonstrate that falls from elevations of 30 feet or less resulted in many ironworker injuries and fatalities. In addition, the Agency recognizes that slips on the same level also lead to many injuries. We believe that provisions to reduce the slip potential of surfaces walked on by steel erection workers are clearly needed. OSHA and SENRAC examined the factors involved in slippery surfaces and determined that the most effective and feasible approach is to increase slip resistance and allow employees to walk on only those coated surfaces which meet a threshold for acceptable slip resistance. Much of the discussion in this rulemaking involves issues regarding which slip-resistant threshold to set; whether it is feasible to measure it; and whether compliance with such a provision is technically and economically feasible.

Commenters affirmed the existence of a serious hazard from coated surfaces; many asserted that slick or slippery paint is very dangerous (Exs. 13–49, 13–66, 13–95, 13–345, 13–348, and 13–355B). Most of these commenters (Ex.13–66 and a group of 124 ironworkers in Ex. 13–355B) added that slippery paint is the worst condition they run into on structural steel, and they asked that the paint be made safe. Other ironworkers (Ex. 13–355B) asserted that epoxy paint was hazardous to erectors. All together, 230 of these ironworkers commented in support of a provision to make painted steel less slippery. A comment from a structural steel fabricator (Ex. 13–228) stated that they agreed that "painted [steel], moist or wet, is slipperier."

In contrast to the comments asserting that coated surfaces present a slipping hazard, a comment from an engineer for a state government agency (Ex. 13–359) stated that slippery surfaces were attributable to a variety of causes, such as weather conditions, which can reduce traction on coated or uncoated surfaces (Ex. 13–359). He added that there was no basis for the requirements that addressed a CoF in subpart R "since there are no accepted methods for determining friction at the job site and tests would not be relevant to site conditions." In addition, the American Iron and Steel Institute Steel Coalition submitted a consultant's report asserting that it is not really necessary to know a CoF in evaluating pedestrian traction, and that it is important to rate the traction under various relevant conditions (Ex. 13–307A, pp. 24–25).

In response to the first concern that slippery surfaces are attributable to a variety of causes, OSHA points out that requiring less slippery coatings in no way suggests that employers should ignore other unsafe conditions. The general construction standard for training/1926.21 requires employers to "instruct each employee in the recognition and avoidance of unsafe conditions ..." This includes slipping hazards due to factors such as moisture from weather conditions and unsafe footwear. OSHA agrees however, with its expert witnesses, William English, David Underwood and Keith Vidal, who stated in their report, that "contaminants" (including rain water, condensation and ice) and shoe bottom construction are important factors, but are not as easily controlled as surface coatings (Ex. 17, p. 2). Also, the rule will require wet testing, thus accounting for most weather-related slip hazards.

In response to the second concern that it is not really necessary to know a CoF in evaluating traction, the final rule text does not set a required CoF — the 0.50 measurement is a slip resistance measurement for the walking surface. While related to CoF (a ratio of forces), the 0.50 referred to in the final rule is a measurement on a tester that is designed to mimic (to some extent) the dynamic forces involved in walking on a surface. While different types of shoe material (and different amounts of wear) affect the amount of traction experienced by the worker, the record shows that it is not feasible to establish a requirement that would account for all the factors that relate to the CoF. Nor would it be feasible to measure slip resistance at the site under the numerous and ever-changing "relevant conditions." The English reports and testimony of English, Underwood and Vidal (as discussed below) shows that setting a requirement for the walking surface (when wet) will improve traction.

A commenter suggested that OSHA focus on ironworkers' footwear rather than specifying a slip resistance for the paint (Ex. 13–307A, pp. 2–5). The Agency finds that this type of approach would not work as a substitute for addressing the slip resistance of the paint because ironworkers' footwear typically become contaminated with mud, gravel, and other substances that would alter the slip resistance characteristics of the sole material (Exs. 203X, p. 213 and 204X, p. 292).

Other commenters recommended that only uncoated surfaces be allowed to be erected (Exs. 13–41, 13–138 through 13–142, 13–234, and 13–341). The record does not demonstrate that uncoated steel is necessary for employee safety since surface coatings can provide equivalent or greater protection against falls. Also, SJI identified several significant problems with requiring the steel to be uncoated when erected. Among these would be increased costs associated with painting the steel in the field after it was erected, which it estimated would amount to $450 to $800 million, and a slowing of the construction process by two to four weeks (Ex. 204X; p.17).

Use of the Term "'Finish Coat"

The final rule specifies the acceptable slip resistance of structural steel "coated with paint or similar material," whereas the proposal limited the provision to steel which had been "finish-coated." This change clarifies that the provision applies to the surface of the coated structural steel when the steel is erected. OSHA believes that the rulemaking record demonstrates that the hazard posed by slippery coated steel is present irrespective of whether the coat is part of a multi-coat system. In addition, we note that both the English I study (Ex. 9–64) commissioned by SENRAC and the English II study (Ex. 17) commissioned by OSHA, which tested slippery coated surfaces, evaluated coatings that were not necessarily "finish" coats. According to Paul Guevin, an OSHA expert witness, the English II study looked at three types of slip-resistant primers: Alkyd paints without additives; zinc-rich primers, and alkyds or other resin-based primers with polyolefin (Ex. 18, p. 2). The modification to "coating" also responds to concerns that it would be difficult to determine which paints are "finish" coats. Thus, the reworded provision now clearly applies to steel members coated with standard shop primers where the shop primer is the uppermost coat when the steel is erected.

A number of commenters asked OSHA to clarify and/or define the term "finish coat" (Exs. 13–182, 13–209, 13–228, 13–363, and 13–367). One of these commenters (Ex. 13–182) opined that finish-coated means painting after erection, which they indicated was done in many situations. A fabricator (Ex. 13–228) commented that a finish coat is the final coat of a multi-coat paint system, whether it was applied in the shop or the field is immaterial. Another commenter (Ex. 13–367, p. 16) noted that "it is frequently not possible to determine if an applied coating is a single coat or a multi-coat system." The American Institute of Steel Construction (AISC) speculated (Ex. 13–209, pp. 31–32) that SENRAC's use of "finish-coat" was an attempt to address certain epoxies and polyurethanes, which are typically the second and third coats found in multi-coat paint systems, but that "[t]he scope of the proposed rule could be twisted to apply to all paints, not merely that small segment of the market that may present a problem." OSHA disagrees with this characterization of the provision's intended application. By deleting the term "finish coat," OSHA clarifies that the provision applies to coated steel on which employees must walk, regardless of whether the coating will remain the last coat of paint after the steel erection is over, and regardless of the chemical composition of the coating.

Benchmark Slip-Resistance Criterion

The final standard requires that coated steel must score at a minimum average slip resistance of 0.50 as measured on an English XL Tribometer or equivalent reading on another tester. Proposed § 1926.754©(3) would have required that the structural steel surface be no more slippery than bare, uncoated steel. OSHA stated in the proposal that SENRAC, after reviewing various industry presentations, "concluded that it could not determine a minimum value for slip-resistance or CoF, given all the variables to be considered, nor could it agree on an acceptable testing method" (63 FR 43468).

After reviewing the entire record, OSHA has determined that it is necessary to set a specific slip-resistance value for coated steel. No other regulatory approach to reducing the risk of slipping is as appropriate. The record supports using the English XL value of 0.50 (or the equivalent) as the cutoff for acceptable coated steel surfaces on which employees may walk. The record demonstrates that acceptable testing methods will be available when the provision goes into effect.

The English II report noted that a level of 0.50 was reasonably safe and has been recognized for many years:

> The non-controversial 0.50 threshold of safety that has been recognized in the safety engineering literature and case law for 50 years would provide a vast enhancement of footwear traction that would produce a significant improvement in the safety of ironworkers working at high elevations. (Ex. 17, p.12)

In post-hearing comments (Ex. 64), Mr. Guevin explained that when the Federal Trade Commission published a proposed rule for floor polishes in 1953 it determined a minimum of 0.50 when measured on a James machine to be a safe value (Ex. 64, pp.3–4). In his testimony at the hearing (Ex. 200X; p.120), Dr. Underwood added that he understood that 0.50 came from rounding up a CoF of 0.35 to give a small margin of safety for walking slowly in a normal way. He indicated that the CoF of

0.35 came from determining a ratio of an average hip height of 3 feet (0.91m) and a common distance of 2 feet (0.61m) per step taken in a normal stride.

The English II study indicates that the recommendation of 0.50 on the English XL scale was based on the previously established benchmark of 0.50 CoF (Ex. 17, p.12). We find that the information and testimony from the rulemaking record show that 0.50 on the English XL scale is an appropriate minimum value to designate slip-resistant surfaces when measured under wet conditions using the ASTM methods referenced in Appendix B to this subpart.

As noted above, OSHA is changing the proposed benchmark for acceptable slip-resistance, from bare steel, to a specific slip resistance value for the coated steel. Thus, there is no need for employers, paint companies or fabricators to measure the slip resistance of bare steel for purposes of complying with this standard. Some participants objected to using the slip-resistance of bare steel as the benchmark. OSHA believes that the revised provision addresses these concerns. A comment from a builder's association (Ex. 13–121) stated that "it is next to impossible to provide CoF equal to original steel after coating it." The Steel Coalition wrote that the proposal's reference to a test for a comparative coefficient of friction in § 1926.754©(c)(3) would not be practical or meaningful, and that coatings with a high slip-resistance score would be considered unacceptable when compared to original steel with a higher score (Ex. 13–307, pp. 35–36). The American Institute of Steel Construction (AISC) (Ex. 13–209, p. 36) stated that "[t]he benchmark of bare steel is ambiguous." AISC explained that using bare, uncoated steel as a benchmark was problematic because it was impossible to find a single uniform steel surface with which to make comparisons — "there is no such thing as a uniform piece of bare steel" (*Ibid,* p. 30). The AISC also objected on the grounds that each piece of steel would have to be tested, before and after it was coated (*Ibid,* p. 30).

The Society for Protective Coatings (SSPC) (Ex. 13–367, p 16) stated that "…data from the English study [English I study] shows that a pristine millscale steel surface received one of the poorest ratings by ironworkers and by the English machine. Therefore, it is extremely risky to make an assumption about slip resistance based on whether the steel is coated or uncoated."

During the hearing, Mr. English testified that he did not support the benchmark of original or bare steel:

> First of all, … pristine bare steel is pretty rare. Secondly, … the baseline would be variable. Thirdly, we find that pristine bare steel, it's slippery … And as a practical matter, it rarely occurs as a problem at erection sites (Ex. 200X; pp.115, 128–129).

Some comments supported using bare steel as the benchmark of acceptable slip-resistance. Journeymen ironworkers (54 individuals, Ex.13–207C) signed statements saying that they backed limiting coatings to the equivalent of bare steel. However they did not provide information concerning the feasibility or adequacy of relying on "bare steel."

In sum, the record supports OSHA's decision that bare steel is not an appropriate benchmark. We agree with the commenters who stated that there is considerable variability in bare steel surfaces due to both manufacturing specifications and extent of oxidation, that variability would also pose substantial problems in implementing the requirement, and that some bare steel is unacceptably slippery.

Test Methods

The final rule requires that beginning three years after the effective date of the rest of the standard, employees may not walk on coated steel unless the coating has been tested and found to meet the threshold 0.50 using an appropriate ASTM test method. Appendix B specifies two methods now approved by ASTM. The record shows that these methods are sufficiently accurate and yield sufficiently reproducible results for use in testing coatings to determine their compliance with the specified 0.50 measurement.

Evidence in the record shows that testing using the VIT (English XL) according to ASTM F1679–96 will provide reproducible and accurate results of the slip-resistance of coated steel: the authors of the English II study stated that the VIT has achieved satisfactory precision and bias according to ASTM E691–92 Standard Practice for Conducting an Interlaboratory Study to Determine the Precision of a Test Method. The report of their testing showed that highly consistent results were produced from repeating the VIT tests, and that there was substantial correlation between the ironworker rankings with VIT rankings.

Also, the final rule's designation of approved ASTM testing methods as appropriate to determine compliance with a performance criterion is consistent with other OSHA standards. For example, in OSHA's standard for nationally recognized testing laboratories, an "ASTM test standard used for evaluation of products or materials" falls under the term "appropriate test standard" (as set out in the introductory text to paragraph (c) of that section, / 1910.7).

Various participants, however, claimed that the two ASTM testing methods lack precision and bias statements, which in their view render those standards "meaningless" (see *e.g.*, Dr. Kyed's testimony Ex. 204X; p. 262 and Ex. 13–367; pp. 3–4). However, various witnesses (including one who offered the position above) stated that precision and bias statements often lagged behind a new approval by ASTM of a test method. "Test methods can be temporarily issued without these statements, but they must eventually comply with this requirement. Generally, it's a 5-year period." (Ex. 204X; p.262). Dr. Mary McKnight from the National Institute for Standards and Technology (NIST), testifying with a panel from the Society for Protective Coating (SSPC) [formerly the Steel Structures Painting Council], agreed that "… within 5 years, there will be a group of laboratories that become proficient in running the test method and who will participate in a round robin study. At the end of this process, ASTM includes a number describing statistical significance of different responses, with a 95-percent repeatability limit and/or confidence level" (Ex. 205X; pp. 56–68). In post hearing comments (Ex. 71, p. 4), Mr. English stated that the ASTM F1679 precision and bias study has been approved by letter ballot, and at a recent meeting of the F13.10 Traction subcommittee, two-thirds of those present voted to find all negatives non-persuasive.

OSHA concludes that the rulemaking record demonstrates that the methods identified in Appendix B are sufficiently reliable in evaluating the slip-resistance of coated steel. The record also shows that this reliability is likely to be confirmed by the ASTM precision and bias statement process within the 5-year period this provision will be delayed.

In posthearing comments, the major industry groups who objected to OSHA's designating ASTM methods stated that "several of their organizations actively participate in research and development efforts involving the validation and adoption of a testing machine and test methodology appropriate to coated structural steel" and recommended that OSHA delay the effective date for 3 years to allow further expert evaluation (Exs. 63, p. 7 and 75, p. 4). These groups also wanted this additional time to determine if implementation of the provision was feasible.

Although the ASTM methods are the best available, OSHA acknowledges that the ASTM methods lack a protocol for representative samples of steel and their preparation. The Agency anticipates that either these parallel issues will be addressed by ASTM within the time frame before paragraph ©(c)(3) becomes final (5 years after the effective date of the final rule) or alternative steps can be taken to ensure accounting for these parameters.

Availability of Paints to Meet the Slip Resistance Benchmark

The final standard delays the effective date of the slip-resistant coating provision for 5 years from the date the rest of the standard becomes effective. This is a change from the proposal, which would not have delayed the effective date. OSHA finds that although some slip-resistant coatings suitable for use in the steel erection industry are now available, widespread distribution and use of suitable coatings will take additional time. We have chosen a 5-year delay in agreement with the post hearing requests of the major organizations commenting on this issue. These organizations submitted their comments as the Unified Steel Construction Consensus Group (USCCG) (Ex. 63), a group that consists of eight large organizations as signatories. The USCCG explained that their membership represents design, engineering, fabrication, manufacturing, and field installation components of the steel construction industry. (The following organizations were listed as signatories: The Steel Joist Institute; Steel Erectors Association of America; National Council of Structural Engineers Associations; National Institute of Steel Detailing; Council of American Structural Engineers; American Institute of Steel Construction; Metal Building Manufacturers Association; and the Society for Protective Coatings.) They stated that the rulemaking record was uncertain about the extent adequate coatings were now available, and that developing, testing and distributing appropriate slip-resistant coatings for the industry would take time. Also, during the rulemaking, many paint formulators and steel fabricators stated that they do not now use the specific paints tested in the English II study. (For example, see Ronner at Ex. 204X, pp. 15 and 108–109; and Appleman at Ex. 205X, pp. 139 and 157–158.) In addition, some formulators and fabricators and their representatives stated that there is a lack of information about whether the paints/coatings in use can meet the standard's slip-resistant threshold. (For example, see Ex. 13–367, pp. 7 and 17; Ex. 13–307, pp. 38–39; Ex. 13–209, pp. 36–37; and Ex. 206X, pp. 34–35.)

OSHA finds that there is some uncertainty as to the extent to which there are adequately slip-resistant coatings currently available that would meet the industry's needs. In view of the fact that there are many such coatings presently on the market (see Ex. 17, pp. 3 and 10–11; Ex. 18, pp. 1–2; Ex. 200X, pp. 54, 62–63, 70, 137–139, and 168–169; Ex. 204X, pp.193–194; Ex. 205X, pp. 139 and 157–158) and the technology for developing additional coatings is in place (see Ex. 205X, pp. 51, 93–94, 99–102, 139, 151–152, 157–158, 167–168 and 217–219; Ex. 63, pp. 3 and 7; and Ex. 64, pp. 2–3), it is reasonable to expect that the 5-year delay will provide enough time for the industry to develop coatings that comply with the final rule.

OSHA agrees that the record evidence on the availability of slip resistant paint which meets the standard is conflicting. The witnesses who conducted the English I study commissioned by SENRAC (Ex. 9–64), and the English II study commissioned by OSHA (Ex. 17), testified that one reason for conducting these studies was to determine whether slip-resistant paint was widely available for use by the steel erection industry. They contended that slip resistant paints are available. They surveyed fabricators first, to identify coatings actually in use for steel erection, tested these coatings in their studies, and found that most of them passed the tests for slip-resistance (Ex.18, pp. 1–2). In post-hearing comments (Ex. 71, p. 4), Mr. English stated that "paints now being applied on something over 80 percent of the fabricated steel products in the U.S. can be easily made to comply with the proposed specification with no complications to application methodology, coatability, corrosion or UV resistance or any of the 'problems' raised by … those opposed to this standard." He added that the paints that do not already comply could be brought into compliance with "the simple addition of the plastic powder …" Another witness (Ex. 205X; pp. 220–221) acknowledged that zinc-rich primers that are currently being used "extensively" had good slip-resistant qualities. However, he also stated that they are not generally used by the industry (*Ibid;* pp. 139 and 157–158).

Various other rulemaking participants told OSHA that the coatings used in the English studies represented only a small percentage of coatings used in steel erection. According to a telephone survey of 180 fabricators conducted by Mr. Ronner for the Steel Joist Institute (SJI) (Ex. 28), only 14 (7 percent) used the paints tested in the English II study (Ex. 204X; p. 15), and that although slip resistant coatings are now used for various military applications such as helicopter flight decks and aircraft carriers, they are not generally used by the steel erection industry (Ex. 205X, pp. 139 and 157–158). The SSPC commented that slip-resistance has not been a design factor for coatings used on structural steel and that slip-resistant paints have not generally been tested for durability (Ex. 13–367, p. 7). A representative of the SJI (Ex. 204X, p. 13) testified that the zinc-rich primers, paint with polyolefin beads and some alkyd-based primers used in the English II study are for spray applications only, are not recommended for dip operations. He added that steel joists typically are coated by dipping them in dip tanks (Ex. 204X; p. 13), and that the industry could not spray on paints due to state and Federal environmental restrictions. These commenters assert that there is no basis for assuming that the same slip resistance would be achieved if the paints were dipped, and that there are technical problems with applying some of the slip resistant paints by dipping. (See for example Mr.

Ronner's testimony, Ex. 204X; p.13, and Mr. Appleman's testimony at Ex.205X; p. 93.) Both Mr. Guevin and Mr. English acknowledged that they do not know if the same slip results reported in the English II study for the paints with beads would be obtained if that paint had been applied by dipping (Ex. 200X; pp. 62–63).

Promising approaches to providing slip-resistant coatings for the steel erection industry were identified during the rulemaking. As explained in the English II study (Ex. 17, p. 11) and as Mr. Guevin (Ex. 200X, p. 56) stated by ICI Devoe in Western Canada developed a slip-resistant 3-coat system, using "DevBeads," an additive of polyolefin beads. However, various participants questioned whether grit particles such as polyolefin beads could be added to paints and primers in steel erection. For example, George Widas (OSHA expert witness who peer reviewed the English II study) questioned whether such coatings would retain their corrosion protection (Ex. 204X; p. 240); Mr. Sunderman of KTA Tator, Inc., questioned whether polyolefins would be degraded by ultraviolet light (Ex. 206X, p. 34–35). Mr. Sunderman also challenged the notion that specific properties of paint can be modified "randomly" without affecting the balance of properties, and without extensive testing and evaluation (Ibid, p. 35–36).

Several participants stated such that slip resistant coatings could be developed for use in steel erection, but that time would be needed to do this. Robert Kogler, a research engineer, explained that testing corrosion control materials takes several years, and they still rely very heavily on long-term exposure data, but are coming up with accelerated testing that gives us reasonable data (Ex. 205X; p. 74, to same effect, see testimony of Dr. Appleman Ex. 205X; p. 51).

On a related issue OSHA finds that obtaining documentation or certification that coated steel meets this requirement also is feasible. However, paint manufacturers told OSHA in their post hearing comments that they will work with interested parties to formulate, test and evaluate coatings to meet the standard's criteria. (See Exs. 63, p. 7 and 75, p. 4 and 205X, p. 218.) Mr. Guevin testified that based on his experience with contacting paint manufacturers to obtain slip-resistant coating for the English II study, and his knowledge of typical paint technical bulletins issued by manufacturers setting out specifications, tests conducted, and results, companies would readily certify if their coatings meet OSHA slip-index requirements in accordance with the recognized ASTM Method (Ex. 200X; p. 168). Thus, OSHA does not agree with a project manager for a steel fabricator (Ex. 13–300) who commented that the requirement was "not viable" because paint manufacturers will not provide documentation out of concerns for liability.

In sum, OSHA finds that although there are slip-resistant coatings in use for structural steel in limited specialized applications, most of them have not been adequately tested to determine whether they comply with the standard and meet the performance needs of other kinds of structures. The coatings industry has committed to develop, test and distribute coatings that comply with this standard in a reasonable time frame. OSHA believes that the hazard of slipping on coated steel is significant; that the paint and fabrication industries feasibly can produce and use coated steel that complies with this provision within the time frame stated in the regulatory text; and in any event, there are now coatings on the market that meet the standard that can be used to some extent even before the widespread production of new slip-resistant coatings. The need for this provision is amply supported in the record. We believe that by issuing a delay of the effective date of this provision the needs of the industries affected by this provision will be met and the long-term safety concerns of the workers who must walk on these surfaces will also be met.

6 Flooring and Tribometry

6.1 INTRODUCTION

Effectively applying tribometry to walkway surfaces requires an understanding of several key concepts. Knowledge of the history and acceptability of historically meaningful thresholds of safety for slip resistance is essential. Operator competency and equipment condition can make the difference between credible test results and incredible ones. An understanding of how and why wear, cleaning, flooring materials, and finishes can affect traction will assist you in weighing these significant variables when coming to conclusions about test results and actions that may be needed to improve the traction of walkway surfaces.

6.2 THE THRESHOLD OF SAFETY

There is much misinformation about thresholds of safety for slip resistance. Contrary to published charts, no generally accepted safe, dangerous, or very dangerous thresholds have been established by any recognized independent authority. The one commonly mentioned level of "acceptable" slip resistance is 0.5.

It can be argued that the 0.5 threshold has been ratified by ASTM (D2047), UL (UL 410), and ANSI (ANSI 1264.2) (see Chapter 5). The 0.5 threshold is based on establishing the merchantability of new flooring-related materials and finishes using the James Machine (see Chapter 3). In the U.S., it is widely referred to in relation to static coefficient of friction (SCOF), while overseas 0.4 is the historically significant number in connection with dynamic coefficient of friction (DCOF).

Currently, the most significant value of slip resistance testing is its ability to determine the extent of an exposure (e.g., potential for pedestrian falls), and as a tool to establish levels of slip resistance by comparative methods. For example:

- Is this floor material or finish more or less slip resistant than others?
- How significantly is slip resistance affected by moisture or other contaminants?
- Is slip resistance stable or deteriorating due to wear?
- How do cleaning methods affect slip resistance?

For a history of the 0.5 threshold, see Chapter 3.

6.3 USES FOR TRIBOMETERS

6.3.1 Problem Identification — Prevention

In order to take corrective action, you must first know the locations of the problems. In combination with a preliminary analysis of losses, slip resistance testing can assist in identifying problem conditions before they produce accidents. Areas that should be considered include those with high traffic, entrance/exit areas, and areas where history indicates problems may exist.

6.3.2 Little or No Prior History

At certain times, loss history cannot be analyzed because this information is unknown or unavailable. Examples include new ventures, the use of new flooring materials, poor prior accident reporting and investigation procedures, and the acquisition of new properties or business units. In such instances, slip resistance testing alone can be instrumental in helping to identify areas of potential concern.

6.3.3 Claims Defense/Documentation

Performing and documenting periodic slip testing on surfaces that may be subject to slip and fall claims, as part of an ongoing prevention program, can be effective in minimizing claim occurrences and costs.

6.3.4 Accident Investigation

Any factual investigation done today can be scrutinized through the legal process of discovery at a later point in time. Because of this, it is essential that all factual investigation support for claims, including slip resistance testing, be as thorough and accurate as possible. Prompt testing of the area in question and clear and concise documentation of the results can be critical in determining whether the floor surface contributed to the accident.

6.3.5 Assessment of Floor Treatment/Cleaning Products and Methods

Slip resistance testing can provide a means of directly comparing the relative effectiveness of current or proposed floor treatments, cleaning products, and cleaning methods upon application and over time.

The systematic approach to selecting an effective floor treatment, or evaluating a cleaning regimen, is a controlled evaluation. Finding the right product is really a process of elimination. Working with a professional will enable you to document the steps that support your flooring recommendation.

1. Develop a list of potential floor treatment products based on the type and use of flooring, and the appropriateness of the treatment for your application.
2. Review the application and maintenance requirements. Methods vary by the type of treatment; some are simple and safe to apply, others require

professionals. Also, you must be able to live with the care and cleaning requirements, and the maintenance needs (frequency of application).
3. Patch test those products on your flooring to further narrow the field. This is best done by a professional who is trained and experienced in the use of the tribometer selected.
4. Conduct a 30-day trial of those products that performed the best out of the box. Monitor the results by remeasuring the slip resistance, determining changes in slip incidents, and listening to feedback from your staff. This will narrow the field to a handful of products, which you should test for an extended period of 90 days or more.

Of course, the bottom line in selecting a floor treatment is a controlled evaluation. Vendors offering a multifaceted set of solutions can be problematic. For example, a vendor might package shoes, floor treatments, signs, and other program elements. Given that *so many changes were made at the same time,* it is difficult to isolate the aspect or aspects of the program had a significant impact from those that were superfluous. *You need to make one change at a time, then evaluate the results of that change.*

6.4 OPERATOR QUALIFICATIONS OF COMPETENCY

It is essential to ensure that designated staff is properly trained in slip resistance testing. Without being able to support the knowledge and ability of staff to operate a slip test device, there is little value in conducting testing at all. The best way to back up staff competency is to have those conducting testing obtain certification, not just to ensure competency on the testing apparatus and protocol, but also on the general subject and factors involved in slip resistance testing. Such certification should consist of two parts:

1. Knowledge, which can be demonstrated by a written self-study program with a final examination
2. Practical application requiring demonstration of the proper use of the test device

Presently, only one test instrument, the variable incidence tribometer (VIT) or English XL, is known to have a manufacturer-approved user certification program, which is administered by the International Safety Academy (http://www.esis.com/rcs/isa/cert.asp).

6.5 EQUIPMENT CALIBRATION AND MAINTENANCE

Most tribometers require some amount of care. Equipment must be calibrated, maintained, and stored per the manufacturer's specifications. This is essential to assuring and defending the integrity of test results.

Depending on the type of apparatus, a wide variety of components may require periodic or ongoing attention. Examples of such maintenance include gauge calibration, joint and valve lubrication, apparatus leveling, tightening of bolts, broken welds, and detection and repair of damaged or bent parts.

It is also advisable to document calibration results, including date, location, method, individual performing work, and test instrument/serial number.

6.6 IDENTIFYING TYPES OF FLOORING AND THEIR PROPERTIES

It is important to be accurate to properly identify types of floor surfaces. The most compelling reason is that each type involves differing maintenance and housekeeping requirements. Knowing the surface composition is also essential to selecting floor treatments, finishes, and cleaners that are effective and will not damage the material.

However, it can often be a challenge to properly identify the composition of flooring materials. Flooring materials can now be produced in one material that closely resembles another. The wide variety of colors, textures, patterns, and styles add to the confusion. Even the descriptive names of flooring materials can be misleading. Further complicating the identification process are opaque finishes that may be applied to the material, masking their true identity. Finally, there may be no one left at a facility where flooring material was installed many years ago, and there is no longer a record of what was purchased.

In one case, a material named as a type of granite was purchased and installed in an establishment serving liquor because granite is not subject to damage due to alcohol or the acidic content of beverages. Later, it was discovered that the material was in fact an acid-etchable black limestone.

However, even knowing the type of material being used is of limited benefit. Consider that even if you knew the class (e.g., resilient, non-resilient) and category (e.g., marble, granite, limestone) of the material, the properties of slip resistance can vary based on the manufacturer due to the processes used and the extent of quality control, as well as by the particular line of product of the manufacturer. In the case of organic materials such as natural stone, the properties of the material can also vary by the source (e.g., country/region, quarry, vein). Consider that in one database of natural stone materials (http://www.graniteland.com) 266 different types of marble and 524 different types of granite are available. Even the properties of individual pieces of tile can vary from one another.

Even with these drawbacks, an understanding of how to identify flooring materials does yield benefits in assuring that maintenance, housekeeping, and finish requirements are suitable, thus maintaining the desired appearance and extending the life of the floor.

6.6.1 Resilient Flooring

Depending on the texture, resilient flooring is generally highly tractive in the dry condition, but often has low slip resistance when wet. Most resilient flooring is produced and sold in role or tile form. By definition, resilient flooring is flexible and pliant material. The following list further defines resilient flooring:

- *Linoleum* is a flexible floor covering made from oxidized linseed oil or a combination of drying oils, wood flour and/or ground cork, resins, and pigment.
- *Asphalt* in 9-in. square tile form is made with fillers, pigments, and fiber (usually asbestos) with a binder. It is a porous surface that becomes brittle over time and is subject to fading and bleeding. It is commonly found in schools and churches.
- *Rubber* is made from synthetic rubber, fillers, and pigments. It is popular because of its softer sound-deadening qualities. It is a very resilient dense surface and often does not require a seal or finish application. It can be sensitive to solvents and high alkaline cleaners, so neutral cleaners and a soft brush should be used when cleaning.
- *Vinyl* is made from vinyl resins (varieties of plastics) and is frequently used with other agents to make vinyl asbestos tile (VAT) and vinyl composition tiles (VCT). Vinyl composition tile (VCT) is estimated to account for two-thirds of total hard surface flooring sold in the U.S. Many have very low slip resistance in their pristine state, requiring users to apply safe floor finishes and use proper cleaning procedures.
  - *Homogeneous Vinyl* is a high-quality tile constructed of 100% vinyl. It is not porous, does not need a sealer, and is more flexible than VCT. It is available in 12-in. squares or sheets and rolls.
  - *Vinyl Composition Tile (VCT)* replaced VAT some years ago and is used commonly in new construction. It is normally made in 12-in. squares. Made of varying ratios of vinyl and filling agents (usually clay), its porosity varies widely. VCT normally comes with a factory coating that must be removed prior to finish application to ensure proper bonding.

6.6.2 Non-Resilient Flooring

The slip resistance of non-resilient flooring materials, which are characterized by their hard, inflexible properties, varies greatly. Compared with resilient flooring, a wider variety of non-resilient flooring is available; non-resilient flooring is one of the more frequently used materials throughout the world.

Non-resilient tile is generally available in any of three states: virgin fired condition, glazed, and non-slip implants. Virgin tile, such as quarry tile, is a relatively slip resistant surface. Glazed tile is generally too slippery for heavy pedestrian areas. Glazed tiles can be manufactured with non-slip implants, but often the glazing negates the benefits of implants. Normally, virgin tile is installed and then sealed, which gives it a ceramic look and a low slip resistance index.

- *Ceramic tile* is a fired mixture of clays — often glazed. Depending on the texture and finish (which can be high-gloss, matt, or abrasive), ceramic tile can perform well or poorly under wet conditions. It is available in sizes ranging from mosaic (1 in.) to 12 in. × 24 in.
- *Quarry tile* is a broad classification for a baked red clay, set in concrete (grout), in 6-in. or 9-in. squares. It is usually deep red in color and left

unglazed. A highly durable surface, quarry tile can perform well in dry and wet conditions when unsealed and untreated. Because it is commonly used in commercial kitchens, however, it is often subject to oil/grease contamination. If not cleaned properly with a strong non-alkaline degreaser, its natural slip resistant properties can quickly degrade.

- *Concrete slab* is a mixture of cement, sand, crushed stone, and water. Installed in paste form, once set it becomes a hard, durable, and porous surface. The degree of slip resistance obtained from concrete depends largely on the method of finish (e.g., smooth trowel, rough brushed, textured, stamped) and the finish (e.g., paint with grit, paint without). *Concrete tile* is also available in varied forms; depending on how it is finished, it can appear similar to natural stone materials.
- *Terrazzo* is an aggregated mix of granite and polished marble chips in poured Portland cement, leveled off to smooth finish. Frequently used in public buildings, terrazzo displays slip resistance properties similar to marble. A very porous surface, terrazzo is listed by the National Bureau of Standards as a high-risk material for stairway treads and has low slip resistance under wet conditions. Some terrazzo is made with non-slip materials added, such as alundum grit. Because adding this material does not alter the appearance of the surface, however, documentation and testing are the only methods of verification.
- Related to terrazzo, *agglomerates* are also marble chips, but are bound in resin and marble dust instead of cement.
- *Marble* is crystallized calcium carbonate, a limestone with properties altered by intense natural pressure and heat. Highly polished marble is also quite tractive in the dry state. Under wet conditions, however, such surfaces (untreated with a slip resistant finish) become hazardously slippery. Marble is often used for more elegant and costly installations and is one of the most common types of stone flooring.
- The slip resistance of marble varies depending on the origin, cut, and wear patterns of the marble floor. Polished marble generally has a relatively low coefficient of friction (COF) value, but, in some cases, can become worn to a higher, safer value. Marble that is located near a street entrance can be roughened by the "grinding" effect of debris on shoes, while marble located in less traveled areas usually becomes highly polished.
- *Other Natural Stones*. Similar to marble, other natural stone surfaces are generally tractive in the dry state, but can become hazardous under wet conditions.
  - *Granite* is an extremely hard rock surface, and is almost always gray in color. It is frequently used in lobbies. Its dull appearance is improved with seal and finish, which also degrades its slip resistance qualities.
  - *Slate* is a blue or dark gray rock in flagstone-type floors found primarily in lobbies and outdoors. It does not polish naturally.
  - *Limestone,* such as travertine, can appear in a wide variety of textures, colors, and designs.

- *Sandstone* includes *bluestone* (a relatively dense sandstone that is aptly named for its tones of blue, green, and purple) and *flagstone*.
- *Wood,* when properly sealed with a urethane or other permanent sealer to prevent moisture penetration, can be coated with one or two coats of floor finish and maintained like vinyl surfaces. Many woods in stained condition can be used as slip resistant floors; however, the application of some sealants, or "oiling" floors, can degrade slip resistance.
- *Carpet* is made of a variety of textiles with heavy jute backing and natural or synthetic fiber piles including wool, polyester, nylon, and others. Carpet is generally considered a slip resistant floor covering, although soaked carpet with a small weave could become slippery.

6.7 FLOOR FINISHES AND THEIR PROPERTIES

In most cases, replacing flooring is not a cost-effective alternative, so other methods of improving the slip resistance qualities of walkway surfaces need to be considered. In general, the goal is to make the surface as slip resistant as possible. This is best accomplished by finding methods to increase surface roughness, while balancing the aesthetic needs of your business.

It is important to note that while some may last for years, no known slip resistant floor treatment is maintenance free. Each requires maintenance, and most require reapplication at some point. Also, the degree to which these products are effective varies dramatically. Whereas some treatments demonstrate an exponential increase in slip resistance, others can actually decrease it (see appendix). Finally, be aware that, in many instances, appearance is affected by treatments. The desirable "high gloss" look can be dulled. This is another reason that testing prospective treatments on a sample (or a small, less trafficked area) prior to a full installation is advisable.

6.7.1 Conventional Floor Finishes

Polishes and waxes have several purposes including:

- Making the floor easier to clean (dirt does not embed into the tile as easily)
- Providing durability to extend the life of the flooring
- Providing a protective coating
- Increasing gloss to improve appearance

A variety of chemicals go into polishes and waxes. They must be balanced because each chemical influences a different property, including gloss, durability, slip resistance, water resistance, black mark, salt, and detergent resistance. Specific ingredients, some of which can counteract another, affect each chemical.

Waxes are no longer made only from natural waxes; synthetics are used more often. However, waxes contain very little wax of either type, but are mostly of polymers with a small bit of wax for truth in advertising.

The more coats of wax or polish applied, the higher the gloss. On average, one gallon provides one coat over an area of 2000 square feet. This provides a coating 1/10,000 of a millimeter thick, which is 1/40 of an inch of the thickness of a coat of paint. Coating fills in the imperfections (including peaks and valleys that would otherwise serve as runoff channels for water and other contaminants), causing them to smooth out.

Industry experts have stated that changes in formulation cannot be made to waxes in order to make them more slip resistant under wet conditions. The only way to do this would be to make the waxes rougher (e.g., by applying a grit), and this would make them substantially less durable and thus impractical.

In addition to floor surfaces, floor finishes also have an impact on the slip resistance of a given surface. Many floor finishes currently on the market are suspended polymers (plastics) that become interlocked when the floor dries, becoming analogous to a sheet of plastic. The slip resistance that a finish is intended to provide can often be found on the container of floor finish used, under "*Performance Specifications*" (stated in terms of SCOF).

This rating must be taken with a grain of salt because the results were usually achieved by using ASTM D2047 (see Chapter 4). How closely the application instructions were followed also affects the results. Contaminants, cleaning, and maintenance can quickly erode the slip resistance of many conventional floor finishes. Factors include insufficient dilution of cleaning compounds, use of inappropriate detergents or floor finishing compounds, inadequate rinsing or burnishing, and settled or tracked-in dirt. Cleaner residue left on an improperly cleaned floor will mix with the newly applied floor finish, destroying much of its water resistance. The only way to verify the actual slip resistance of the treated surface is to conduct testing.

6.7.2 "Slip Resistant" Floor Coatings

Slip resistant coatings, consisting of an adhesive base material with slip resistant material (usually grit) mixed in or sprinkled on after the base is applied, may be used in specific areas to increase traction on slippery surfaces. Grit mixed into the paint or treatment is preferred. Adding grit after the treatment has been applied is generally less effective because it is less likely to adhere, and is more easily dislodged while in use. This can create a greater hazard, similar to spreading sand on a smooth surface.

Three frequently used abrasive grits are aluminum oxide, silicon carbide, and quartz. Aluminum oxide wears well and does not break easily. Silicon carbide has similarly effective wear qualities, but tends to be brittle and can become less effective when subject to high traffic. Abrasive grit flooring is often coated with polyurethane to make cleaning easier.

Coatings may be brushed, troweled, rolled, mopped, or sprayed on, depending on the individual product, and are available for most types of hard walking surfaces.

6.7.3 Surface Grooving and Texturing

Shallow grooves and textures can be ground into existing concrete, asphalt, slate, marble, granite, and tile floors to increase traction. In grooving, diamond saw blades produce precision cuts at specified depths, widths, and spacing. Grooves help to drain liquids off the walkway to improve slip resistance. The direction of the grooves controls the direction of drainage. The saw blades are positioned close to each other for texturing and produce a surface with a ribbed appearance.

Unless cleaned properly, grooving and etching may not be an effective long-term solution. These processes (by cutting into the surface) may result in leaching of contaminants (such as grease and oil) into the surface. Even alkaline-based cleaners and degreasers leave deposits and residues in grooves that can gradually reduce surface slip resistance, with the potential for making slip resistance worse than if no treatment had been applied at all. Cleaning grooved surfaces can be a challenge. Grooving is more commonly used for hard, exterior surfaces such as brick and stone.

6.7.4 Etching

Etching treatments contain diluted hydrofluoric acid or other acidic solution, which creates micro-grooves in the floor surface, thus roughening it to increase slip resistance. The treatment is applied, and a water rinse is used to stop the etching process. The degree of slip resistance depends on the strength of the acid solution applied to the surface and the length of time it is applied. Due to the hazardous nature of the chemicals involved and the importance of proper application, most etching treatments require installation by trained professionals.

Typically, the stronger the solution (and higher the slip resistance), the less glossy is the surface. You may need to experiment with samples to get the right balance of gloss and slip resistance.

Etching can be effective on smooth, hard walkway surfaces such as stone/hard mineral surfaces and agglomerates (resin-based rock products). Vendors may have different formulations for different types of floor surfaces.

Because this treatment involves the removal of some amount of the floor surface material, it can decrease the service life of the flooring. Treatments can last for years. Vendors have guarantees ranging from one to ten years; however, proper cleaning must be performed in order to avoid accumulation of contaminants. In most cases, any commercially available cleaner/degreaser will do, as long as the surface is well rinsed.

6.7.5 Other "Slip Resistant" Floor Treatments

Other treatments are designed to create a raised texture with the use of abrasive crystals, which are bonded to the surface. Such topical coatings can be so dense as to inhibit adherence to the surface, thus requiring more frequent maintenance and reapplication than other types of treatments. Also, keep in mind that some coatings will not properly adhere to polished stone, porcelain, or similar surfaces.

Some treatments are a hybrid of coating and etching. Hydrofluoric acid can be used to soften the grit to improve adherence to the floor surface.

In general, coatings and other similar treatments can deteriorate more quickly than etching and grooving due to wear and cleaning.

6.8 THE IMPACT OF WEAR

Flooring materials in service will wear. Usually, continued use will "polish" the surface, thereby reducing its slip resistance. This is due to the wearing down or smoothing of the asperities in the surface, or the micro-peaks in the material that establish its roughness.

Directionality of surface roughness is also a factor to be considered in slip resistance measurement. Asperities become smoother in the direction of travel as the peaks are worn down and rounded. Thus, a surface may demonstrate greater slip resistance when traversing the area in a direction not normally crossed. Likewise, surfaces with a directional pattern or grain may exhibit different slip resistance properties depending on the direction of travel.

6.9 CLEANING METHODS

The quality and quantity of the following components help determine the effectiveness of a cleaner:

- *Solvency* – Ability to dissolve the material it contacts
- *Emulsification* – Ability to break down a liquid into particles and suspend them in liquid
- *Surfaction* – Ability to lower surface tension and speed up solvency and emulsification
- Surface tension is the tendency of water to bead up, which retards surface wetting and inhibits cleaning. Surfactants are classified by their ionic (electrical charge) properties in water: anionic (negative charge), nonionic (no charge), cationic (positive charge), and amphoteric (positive or negative charge). Soaps are anionic surfactants, made from fats and oils (or their fatty acids) by chemically treating them with a strong alkali.

The effectiveness of soaps lessens when used in hard water. Water hardness is the result of mineral salts that react with soap to form soap film.

6.9.1 Types of Floor Cleaners

Alkaline cleaners are designed to react with fats and oils, converting them into soap (saponification). To remove this slippery residue, the floor must be thoroughly rinsed with clean, hot water. It cannot be permitted to dry; otherwise polymerization can occur (see Section 6.9.4, Traditional Cleaning).

Acidic cleaners use a process called oxide reduction instead of saponification to remove contaminants, and thus polymerization cannot occur.

Neutral cleaners are typically used on glossy floor finishes, or those that can be dulled by the abrasive qualities of alkaline or acidic-based cleaners. These are usually relatively free-rinsing.

High-pH cleaners may be needed to remove grease stains, while acidic chemicals may be needed for mineral buildup from hard water or lime deposits. For daily maintenance, neutral cleaning chemicals are generally recommended. Acids and high-pH cleaners can scar hard floor surfaces (such as marble, terrazzo, and other natural stones).

6.9.2 Floor Finish Condition Indicators

Indicators of a floor finish in poor condition include:

- Spills cannot easily be removed without leaving a stain.
- The floor has a yellow, gray, or patchy appearance (indicating wax buildup).
- The floor finish is flaking or chipping.
- The floor has a visibly dull finish with dark "wear" spots.
- Bare floor shows through the finish/sealer.
- When burnishing, the floor pad quickly becomes dirty.

6.9.3 Mopping Issues

When a mop solution (water containing detergent) is applied, it emulsifies the soil, and releases it from the surface. While suspended in the solution, the loosened soil should be easily removed by the mop, transferred to the rinse bucket, and discarded. If pickup is incomplete, the soil-laden solution settles into low spots on the floor (including grout lines and in the textured "valleys" of floor surfaces). The water evaporates, leaving a residue of detergent and soil particles that attaches firmly to the surface. Over time, if this cycle of incomplete cleaning is repeated, soil and detergent buildup becomes substantial and visible, especially when wet. Continuing such "slop mopping" can result in spreading this buildup to the remainder of the floor area.

6.9.4 Common Cleaning Scenario

Typically, major floor-cleaning jobs are performed at night when traffic is lightest. Unfortunately, the low priority placed on floor cleaning results in cost cutting, which impacts the quality of the job. Whether the work is performed in-house or by an independent contractor, a common scenario involves workers, who are hired at low wages with minimal supervision, using the least expensive cleaning supplies and poorly maintained equipment.

Typically, floors are cleaned by first dust mopping (or dry mopping) and then wet mopping. This process works better in theory than in practice. In theory, a clean, freshly treated dust mop is first used to remove dry contaminants including loose debris, grit, and soil. In reality, the condition of the mop is often such that it deposits more contaminants than it removes. Disposable dust mops are available, but there is a tendency to overuse them due to the expense involved. Mop cleaning should be available, optimally by either an open hose on a vacuum or (preferably) in a washing machine.

In theory, the worker next obtains a new or cleaned mop head with a fresh pail of water/cleaner and begins mopping up to the square foot area specified by the floor cleaning product cleaner. Then, the mop is cleaned or changed, and the pail is cleaned and filled with fresh water and cleaner. In practice, workers usually fill a bucket once, use the water mixed with cleaning solvent to swab an area far larger than recommended by the manufacturer of the cleaner, and use a dirty mop. The result is that the solvent loses effectiveness, becoming diluted and increasingly contaminated. The end result is that dirt, grease, and contaminants that may have been confined to one small section are spread over a much wider area.

It has been demonstrated that, within about a month of continuous mopping in oil or grease-laden environments (e.g., restaurants, supermarkets), a hard, clear, shiny layer forms. Although the floor is still slip resistant under dry conditions, traction becomes lower when the floor is wet. This phenomenon is known as polymerization, in which the oils break down into fatty acids that attach to the surface, making them difficult to dislodge through cleaning by mopping (non-agitation) methods.

Polymerization is defined as "the process of chaining together many simple molecules to form more complex molecules with different physical properties which combine and harden. The changing of a compound into a polymeric form by this process." This results in a film that is impervious to detergents at warm and moderately hot temperatures.

Although mopping is not as effective as agitation, effective approaches to floor cleaning with the use of mops are available. A better procedure begins with removal of loose soil and other particle debris by vacuuming and/or sweeping first. Next, a detergent solution can be applied with a clean mop. Finally, after allowing the solution time to penetrate and loosen the dirt, the dirt can be removed with a clean mop and deposited into a bucket of clean rinse water.

6.9.5 Agitation

Mopping is simply not a viable method for removing a polymerized surface. An effective solution is to use a deck brush or automatic scrubbing equipment, with water of 160°F or higher, followed by wet vacuuming or comparable removal of residue prior to rinsing. Although it may require more effort, and perhaps more time, the agitation created by scrubbing cleans the walkway surface far more thoroughly than does mopping. This approach is strongly recommended for high-traffic areas that become extremely slippery when wet or frequently become contaminated. An additional benefit of automatic scrubbing is that fresh water and soap is continuously applied and moves aside the used solvent, thus providing optimal cleaning conditions.

6.9.6 Porous and Sealed Floor Surfaces

The natural surface porosity of a porous floor surface gives the floor its slip resistant characteristic. Over time, these pores become blocked, causing the floor to be more slippery. Organic and inorganic causes of pore blockage must be removed to achieve a safer floor. Traditional cleaners and degreasers can adequately remove fats, oils, grease, and solid deposits, but not inorganic stains.

The problem is different on sealed floors. Traditional cleaners may succeed in degreasing sealed floors. But to achieve safer floors, the floors must be effectively cleaned and provided with a slip reducing agent.

6.9.7 Texturing

The type and amount of texturing can have a major impact on cleaning. Higher-profile texturing presents a greater challenge to thorough cleaning. Eventually, the buildup of contaminants and the wear of the texturing can negate the benefits of texturing. Cleaning on flooring with smaller grit sizes is usually easier than larger grits.

6.9.8 Other Maintenance Issues

Some maintenance issues that should be considered when establishing an effective floor maintenance program include:

- Soil impregnation is soil trapped in the finish. To remove this embedded dirt, the wax/polish coat must be removed and reapplied. Burnishing can further embed the dirt, which is why the floor needs to be cleaned well in the first place (e.g., dry mop, wet mop, applying cleaner, reapply finish).
- The polish film can get "cut," which is difficult to properly clean as the dirt goes deep into the film. Cleaning needs to go beyond the standard procedure to effectively remove dirt embedded into a cut.
- Scuffmarks abrade the coating, leaving a rough surface. The more wax is applied, the less scuffing occurs because the wax coating absorbs the energy of the heel strike.
- High-speed burnishing removes some porting of the coating by abrading some of the film. Continuous burnishing without reapplying polish can result in thin or no coating left.
- Spray buffing is often used in institutional settings (e.g., schools and hospitals) to soften the finish; however, spray buffing also removes layers of material.

6.10 MAINTENANCE AND CONDITION OF FLOOR CARE EQUIPMENT

The quality of the treatment and cleaning of floor surfaces is dependent not only on the chemicals and procedures in use, but also the maintenance of the floor care equipment and supplies. The following are some general guidelines and best practices for these tools:

Dust Mops
- Do not use on wet, oily floors.
- Hang up the mop, with the head down and not touching the floor, when not in use.
- When soiled, the mop head should be changed.
- Be sure that the mop block or frame is the proper size for the mop head.

Floor Machines
- Rest the machine on its wheels, not on its brush or pad driver.
- Clean the machine and the electrical cord after each use.
- Regularly inspect the cord for fraying or loosening.
- It is safest to wear rubber overshoes and rubber gloves when operating on a wet floor.
- Check on nuts, bolts, or screws that may become loose.
- Only qualified personnel should perform motor adjusting or repair.

Mop Bucket and Wringer
- Keep screws and bolts tightened.

- Keep casters properly lubricated and in good repair, and replace them when necessary.
- Clean both the bucket and wringer after each day's use. Too much force on the wringer can break it; do not lengthen the handle.
- Make sure the bucket and wringer are large enough for mop that is being used.
- Remove loose mop strands and other articles caught in the wringer.

Push Brooms

- Rotate the brush frequently so as not to unduly wear one side.
- Do not lean heavily on the handle.
- Do not let the brush stand on the fibers because this will bend them out of shape and make the brush useless.
- Use the broom only for the purposes intended, never as a mop, squeegee, lever, or hammer.
- Be sure you have a large enough brush for the job.
- Combing the brush every week or so will keep it in best operating condition.

Wet Mops

- Do not twist or squeeze the mop too hard because this will break the strands.
- When in storage, do not let wet mops touch other equipment.
- Be sure that the wet mop is rinsed and wrung after each use.
- Be careful when using the mop on splintered floors or floors with projecting nails, so as to not catch and tear the strands.
- Economy of effort dictates that worn mop heads should be replaced.
- When storing mops, hang them up so that they do not touch the floor and the strands do not touch the wall.

6.10.1 Preventative Maintenance Check for Floor Machines

Appearance

- Machine body is clean.
- Bump wheels and splashguards are operational.

Water System

- Solution tank is clean.
- Filter screens are clean.
- Water valves are operational.
- Water hoses are in good repair.

Recovery System Vacuum

- Vacuum heads are clean.
- Recovery tank is clean.
- Machine hood is raised.
- Tank gaskets are dry.
- Drain system is operational.
- Squeegee is clean, and squeegee assembly is operational.

Drive System Wheels
- Front and rear wheels are greased.
- Brush pressure arm is greased.
- Pivot points are oiled.
- Brushes are clean, dry, and in good repair.
- Pad holders are operational, and the pad is the proper size.

Electrical System
- Switches are operational.
- Wiring is in good repair.
- Vacuum and drive motors are clean.
- Batteries
  - Water level is correct (check weekly and refill as necessary using distilled water but do not overfill).
  - Posts and tops are clean.
  - Charger and connectors are operational.
  - Batteries are charged.
  - Batteries are stored in dry, cool places, but above 32°F.

6.11 FLOOR TREATMENT STUDY

In an extensive study, ESIS, Inc. evaluated ten floor treatments, which clearly demonstrated the wide range of effectiveness of treatments marketed as slip resistant. There are a host of reasons why the names of the products have not been released:

Unfortunately, there is no "silver bullet" for slip resistance. The problem is that each situation is different. The study determined only that the treatments tested did indeed work (or did not work), out of the box, on new (unworn and uncontaminated) marble and ceramic tiles. This does not indicate how these products will perform in the presence of various contaminants, under worn conditions, or on other types of flooring. The study was trying to point out that, even under identical conditions, floor treatments vary right out of the box. When you add in significant variables, such as wear, contaminants, and types and grades of flooring, you can not come to any conclusions.

Other concerns are application and maintenance. Some of these treatments require professional application and use caustic chemicals. Some require more frequent cleaning and reapplication than others.

All these issues come down to the fact that each situation needs to be evaluated individually. There is no "one size fits all" situation. What will work for one facility may not be appropriate for another. A treatment that works great in water situations may be terrible in greasy situations. A treatment that is great on marble may be terrible on vinyl. In fact, a treatment that is highly effective on one grade, type, or manufacture of marble may not be as effective on another.

EXHIBIT 6.1
SLIP RESISTANT TREATMENT STUDY 2000

ESIS Risk Control Services

Slip Resistant Treatment

Study 2000

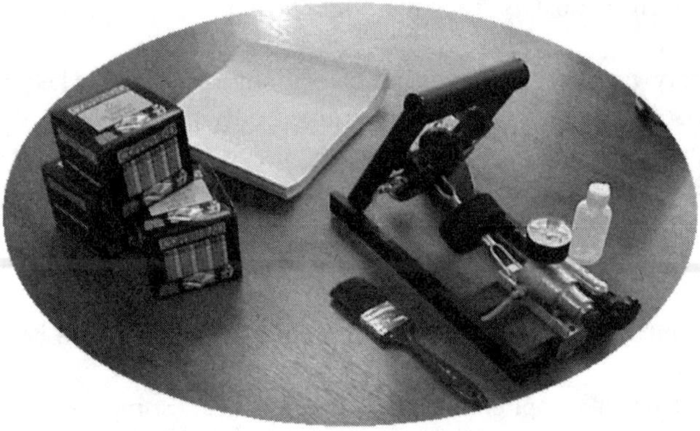

One of the ACE Group of Companies

ESIS Risk Control Services

Slip Resistant Treatment Study 2000

Table of Contents

ESIS Risk Control Services

Slip Resistant Treatment Study 2000

Introduction

This study represents a refinement of earlier research completed in 1998. Both studies, however, were conducted in response to our loss control clients' need to develop a more proactive or solutions-oriented approach to reducing their slip and fall risk.

There are currently hundreds of floor surface treatment products on the market that claim to provide slip resistance. The true efficacy of these products – apart from the manufacturers' claims – is, however, unknown.

Most products tested provided some improvement in slip resistance. Others offered a dramatic improvement. In some cases, resistance was actually reduced. Overall, effectiveness varied widely, particularly on wet test surfaces.

The results offer the first clear evidence from a scientific study that noteworthy differences among slip resistance floor treatment products do exist. They also suggest that manufacturers' product information may not be a reliable guideline in selecting the right products to assist in reducing slip and fall loss costs.

Slip and fall accidents account for a majority of general liability claims in real estate, financial and retail operations. They also represent the second most frequent type of occupational injury. Their causes and control are therefore critical to successful loss control.

The study findings are not intended as opinions on the quality, merchantability, or fitness for the intended purpose of any product. Neither ESIS nor the authors of the study express any opinion on whether any products are defective in any way, and the study draws no conclusion, inference or implication that any product is in any way dangerous, defective or manufactured or designed improperly. No opinion is intended or offered with respect to the adequacy of any product warning.

Goals

The goal of this study was to compare the relative effectiveness of a variety of slip resistance floor treatment products.

This study was conducted for the purpose of increasing the existing body of knowledge among safety professionals concerning a particular type of safety hazard. All findings are relative only in that all comparisons are between and among the products tested. No opinions are offered with respect to any product not tested.

Overview

Two types of floor surfaces were selected for testing. Test surfaces were (1) glazed ceramic tile and (2) marble in 12" x 12" squares, purchased at a retail facility.

A number of slip resistance floor treatment product manufacturers were contacted and invited to participate. The ten (10) vendors who agreed to be a part of this study are identified as Group One through Group Ten.

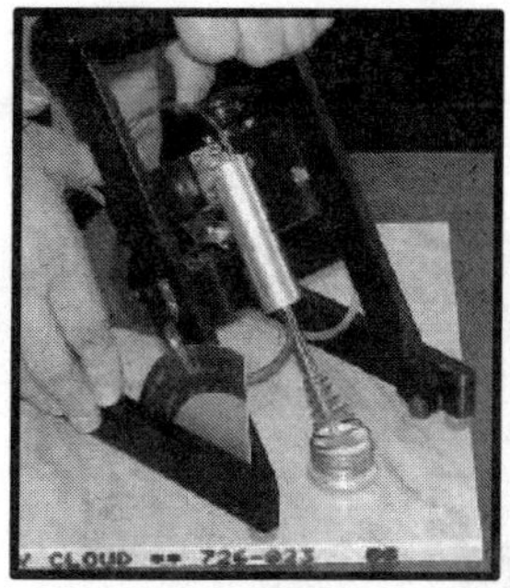

Each set of two surfaces was pre-tested as indicated below. One set of surfaces for each vendor was packed and shipped via UPS with instructions regarding application, documentation, and return transit.

Once the treated surfaces were returned to ESIS RCS from the vendors, they were re-tested under the same conditions. The results were recorded and compared. David Underwood, Ph.D., an analytical chemist and member of the American Society for Testing and Materials (ASTM) technical committee F-13, performed the statistical analysis. ASTM F-13, *Safety and Traction for Footwear*, develops standards and methodologies for slip resistance testing. Dr. Underwood compared the results obtained during pre-testing with those obtained from the treated tiles.

Protocol

The test instrument for this study was a Variable Incidence Tribometer [VIT], which was inspected and calibrated by the manufacturer prior to pre-testing and again prior to the testing of treated tiles. The English XL has undergone a series of "round robin" workshops, conducted by the American Society for Testing and Materials (ASTM) over several years to demonstrate repeatability and reproducibility of test results.

The test foot material for this study was Neolite® test liner*, a generic and durable substance that is one of the most commonly used materials for slip resistance testing. Unlike leather, the properties of which are affected by moisture and wear, the characteristics of Neolite test liner do not change under normal conditions. Neolite test liner is recommended by the tribometer manufacturer, and specified by ASTM D-5859, *Standard Test Method for Determining the Traction of Footwear on Painted Surfaces Using the Variable Incidence Tribometer*.

Testing was done in accordance with:

- *ASTM F-1679 Standard Test Method for Using a Variable Incidence Tribometer* (VIT), released in 1996, which recognizes the English XL VIT as a valid slip resistance field testing device for wet and dry surfaces.
- The most recent release (updated June 1999) of the instruction manual and supplement published by the manufacturer for the English XL Slip Resistance Tester.
- The test foot preparation protocol was done in accordance with the manufacturers' current specifications, using 180 grit silicon carbide sandpaper.

*Neolite® is a registered trademark with Goodyear Tire and Rubber Company.

Other Specifications

Pre-testing and treated testing were completed at a single location, in a temperature-controlled environment, and on the same level surface. Treated tile testing was performed on the same portions of the test quadrants identified and tested during pre-testing. All testing was completed by the same operator, a member of ASTM F-13 and F-06 (*Resilient Floor Coverings*) who is ESIS-certified in slip resistance testing and has five (5) years of experience with the tribometer.

For statistical reliability, three sets of four readings (one for each quadrant) were taken.

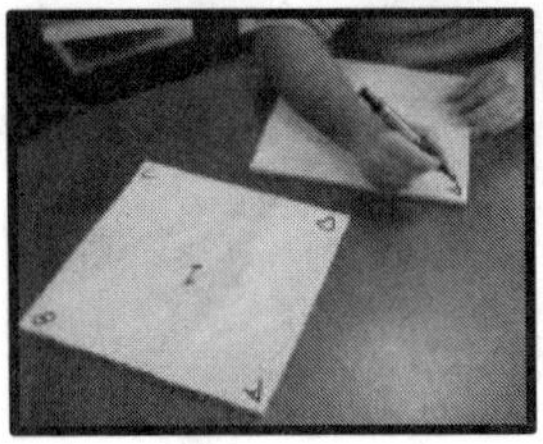

Surface Preparation

Each surface was marked using an indelible marker on the underside of each tile, indicating:

- testing quadrant (A, B, C, D)
- group number (1B10)

The tiles were cleaned by running them through a dishwasher, and were allowed to air dry.

Test Notes

- Tested each quadrant dry, then each quadrant wet
- Completed all dry testing for all surfaces first, then performed wet testing

Dry Testing		**Wet Testing**	
Relative Humidity	*39% - 42%*	*Relative Humidity:*	*41% - 43%*
Temperature (F):	*75° - 77°*	*Temperature (F):*	*72°*

Packing & Shipping

Each group (set of two pre-tested tiles) was packed and shipped to vendors in the following manner:

- Each tile was packed with three layers of bubble wrap, secured with cellophane packing tape
- A layer of packing "peanuts" was placed at the bottom of the shipping carton
- A layer of packing peanuts was placed between the tile packages and on top of the last tile to the top of the box
- Shipping was done by UPS ground transportation
- The tiles were returned by the same method shipped (UPS Ground Ship – prepaid)
- Return packaging used the same method and materials (e.g., bubble wrap and box) as the outgoing shipment
- Condition of packing and tiles upon receipt was good: no visible damage was noted

ESIS Risk Control Services

Slip Resistant Treatment Study 2000

Comparison of Results - Ceramic

Ceramic – Dry

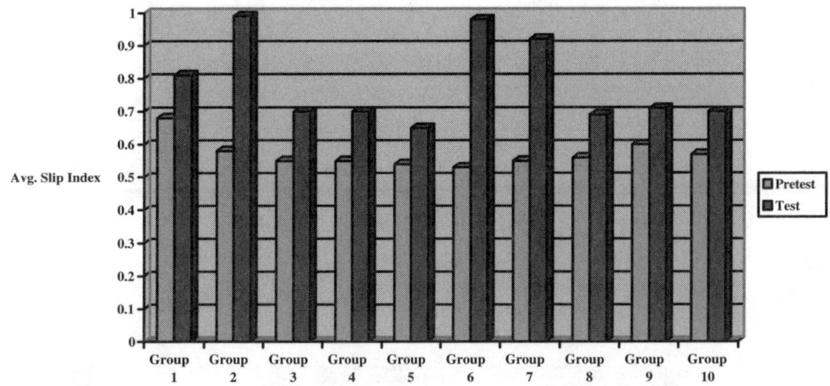

On dry ceramic, even the untreated tiles exceed the generally recognized 0.50 guideline. While all treatments increased slip resistance to some degree, some treatments (such as Groups 2, 6, and 7) provided substantial improvement, exceeding 0.9.

Comparison of Results - Ceramic

Ceramic – Wet

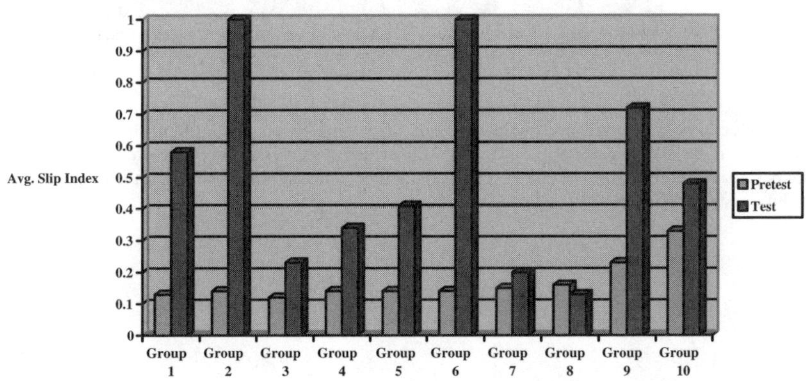

Wet ceramic untreated tiles were mostly between 0.1 and 0.2 X very low slip resistance. All but one treatment (Group 8, which actually decreased) increased slip resistance, and Groups 1, 2, 6, and 9 provided improvement beyond 0.50. Additionally, Groups 2 and 6 did not slip, even at 1.0, the most horizontal position of the tribometer. This is a remarkable result, since both treatments managed to increase slip resistance from approximately 0.1 to more than 1.0, a ten-fold improvement.

Comparison of Results - Marble

Marble – Dry

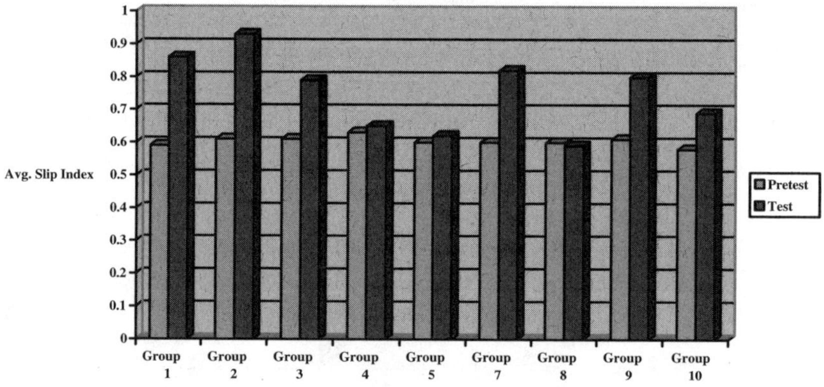

Like dry ceramic, untreated dry marble exceeds the generally recognized 0.50 threshold. While some treatments (such as Groups 1, 2, and 7) provided the most improvement (exceeding 0.8), others showed minimal improvement (Groups 4 and 5), and one demonstrated an actual decrease in slip resistance (Group 8).

Comparison of Results - Marble

Marble – Wet

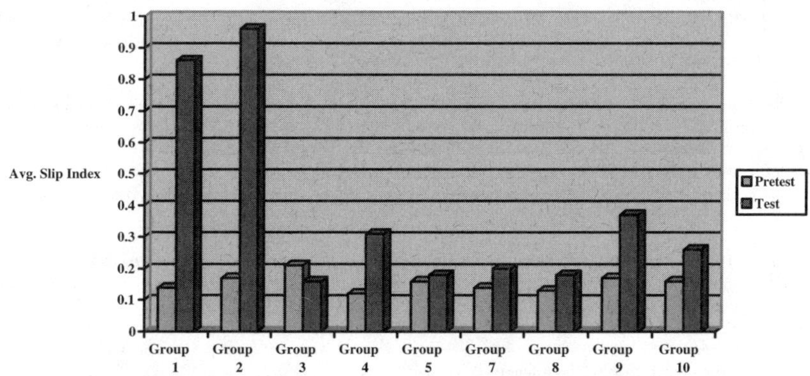

Wet marble untreated tiles pre-tested in a way similar to wet ceramic, mostly in the 0.1 to 0.2 range. It is clear that Group 1 and 2 treatments demonstrated dramatic improvements (beyond 0.8 and 0.9 respectively). Others, such as Group 5, 7, and 8, showed minimal increases. The Group 3 treatment showed a reduction in slip resistance from the untreated condition of the wet marble.

Note: Group 6 was omitted from marble results, since no testing was performed.

ESIS Risk Control Services
Slip Resistant Treatment Study 2000

Credentials and Claims*

The product information available on products falls into one of two primary categories. Some vendors advertise that their products will meet or exceed applicable federal laws. Many state they meet industry consensus standards by engaging an independent testing firm or by testing the product in-house. In comparing the claims of vendors against the study results, there appeared to be low correlation between product claims and the efficacy of the product.

*The information for this section was gathered from additional and prior research, and is not limited to the vendors that participated in this study.

Federal Laws and Standards

The two most cited federal laws with regard to slip resistance are from the Occupational Safety and Health Administration (OSHA) and the Americans with Disabilities Act (ADA). Some vendors claim to meet or exceed the "standards" or "requirements" contained within these laws.

The OSHA "standard" for slip resistance is not a law, nor is it a standard. It is a proposed non-mandatory appendix item set by OSHA and was never adopted as a standard (it specifies slip resistance of 0.50 or higher for the workplace). While it is possible for an OSHA inspector to cite this guideline under the "General Duty Clause," we could find no evidence that this is done in practice. What makes this particularly difficult is that OSHA has specified no test protocol or device upon which to base a citation X effectively making it unenforceable.

The ADA "law," like OSHA, is also a guideline, since the specification appears in an appendix. And because no test protocol or device is specified, even this recommendation is difficult to apply. The ADA specifies slip resistance of at least 0.60 for level surfaces and 0.80 for ramps, where accessible by persons with disabilities. Subsequent to enactment of the ADA, it was determined that the study conducted to validate the specified level of slip resistance was faulty. The study used a laboratory force plate to measure traction demand for the handicapped.

The Architectural and Transportation Barriers Compliance Board (also known as the ATBCB or Access Board) of the U.S. Department of Justice was created to ensure federal agency compliance with the Architectural Barriers Act (ABA). The Access Board adopted the ADA recommendations, and has stated these specifications as a guideline, not a requirement or a standard. Again, no test protocol (e.g., device or test method) is specified.

Consensus Standards

Meeting or exceeding a consensus standard is another often-cited feature in the advertising of slip resistance floor treatments. In some cases, these standards provide only a testing methodology, not a measure of safety; in others, the test method of a standard is modified or not followed properly. Finally, the standards themselves may be obsolete.

American Society of Testing and Materials (ASTM)

The ASTM is the most active organization in the development of standards for measuring slip resistance. The ASTM has promulgated standards for a number of tribometers, including the Variable Incidence Tribometer (VIT or English XL) and the Portable Inclineable Articulated Strut Slip Tester (PIAST or Brungraber Mark II).

However, with the exception of Standard D-2047 (involving a specification of 0.5 for the James Machine – see UL below), the ASTM has never offered a slip resistance threshold of safety, making it impossible to "exceed" an ASTM slip resistance standard. Most ASTM standards are "test methods," or steps to follow in arriving at a measure of slip resistance. "Meeting" an ASTM test method standard only means that the proper steps were followed using the appropriate test device. It is not relevant to the results of the testing, just to the method of reaching those results.

Tests to demonstrate the effectiveness of a treatment are often done using a horizontal dynamometer pull-meter method, a device requiring the use of a 50-pound weight. It is known by experts for overestimating the slip resistance of wet surfaces due to a phenomenon known as "sticktion." This ASTM document, *Standard Test Method for Determining the Static Coefficient of Friction of Ceramic Tile and Other Like Surfaces by the Horizontal Dynamometer Pull-Meter Method* (C1028) has not been updated in many years. In addition, ensuring proper design and calibration of a self-constructed instrument brings into question the validity of the results.

One vendor cited ASTM D-56 in relation to the slip resistance qualities of the product. ASTM D-56 is titled *Standard Test Method for Flash Point by Tag Closed Tester*, and is not related to slip resistance.

Ceramic Tile Institute (CTI)

Some vendors will market a slip resistance floor treatment on the strength of meeting or exceeding requirements as required by the Ceramic Tile Institute (CTI), an industry group representing the interests of the ceramic tile industry. CTI specifies use of ASTM C1028, which is a test method only and does not specify a level of safety. C1028 cannot be exceeded, since it specifies no "safe" or "unsafe" level of slip resistance.

Underwriters' Laboratories (UL)

Many vendors state that their products are classified or certified by Underwriters' Laboratories (UL) as to slip resistance.

While UL does not "certify" products as to slip resistance, it does "classify" products as such. UL will apply the treatment to a surface and test it to UL 410, using the James Machine. To qualify for classification and be permitted to use the UL Classification Marking, test results must show a slip resistance of greater than 0.50, and the manufacturer must pay a fee. Documentation of classification does not provide actual test results, but states only that it was greater than the minimum of 0.50.

The James Machine is a laboratory device designed to test under ideal conditions only for merchantability (the suitability of the product for sale) of new flooring products. This standard is inappropriate for application for field testing.

The James Machine is a complex device for which there are still no standard set-up, operating procedures, or precision and bias from any independent laboratory or consensus standards-making organization.

Complicating the situation, there have been several manufacturers of this device, and in each instance the apparatus was designed and built somewhat differently. Most important, the James Machine is not designed (or even listed by UL) for wet testing. Thus, testing done using this device can be considered questionable.

Independent Laboratory Testing*

The use of independent laboratories for testing products is a frequent component of marketing for slip resistance floor treatments. In most cases, these laboratories use the ASTM or UL standards. However, information demonstrating that the laboratory is qualified to perform such specialized testing is rarely available, and details on the conditions and results of testing are likewise unavailable.

*The examples used in this section are not quotes from any specific product or vendor, but are intended to illustrate the types of claims a consumer may have to interpret.

Example:
... the increase in friction of wet surfaces was between 150% to 500%, based on independent testing with the James Machine.

Aside from the lack of details on the testing, the James Machine is not designed (or listed by UL) for wet testing, making these results irrelevant.

Example:
... tested by one of America's leading independent testing laboratories ... results exceeded all national standards for dry floors, with a 300% increase on wet ceramic tile and 100% on wet marble.

Again, testing was done using the James Machine, inappropriate for all but dry laboratory testing of pristine surface materials. And while our tests also showed a 300% increase in ceramic tile when wet, our results showed 0.41, still below 0.50, the generally recognized safety level of slip resistance. For wet marble, our testing did not show an increase of 100%, but of 12.5%.

Example:
... thoroughly tested and approved by an independent testing laboratory.

The testing laboratory is a provider of insurance and financial services to automotive-related businesses. No details of test device, protocol, and results were provided.

Example:
Independent testing was done in 1993 in accordance with ASTM C1028.

Aside from the age of this testing, the testing laboratory specializes in providing environmental and geo-technical consulting services, and does not appear to have expertise in slip resistance testing.

Conclusions and Summary

The measurement of slip resistance is an emerging field. New technology that was unavailable 10 years ago has pushed reliability far forward. But, it is essential that consensus organizations like the ASTM continue to oversee and refine standards and practices in slip resistance. At the same time, there needs to be a more sophisticated awareness about how current standards and technology might be applied appropriately, as well as their limitations.

With regard to slip resistance floor treatments, it is clear that more work needs to be done in evaluating the efficacy of these products. Hopefully, the results of this study will help demonstrate the wide range in effectiveness, as well as what is involved in interpreting marketing approaches used by manufacturers of these products.

ESIS Risk Control Services

Slip Resistant Treatment Study 2000

Exhibit: Test Protocol

Test Preparation

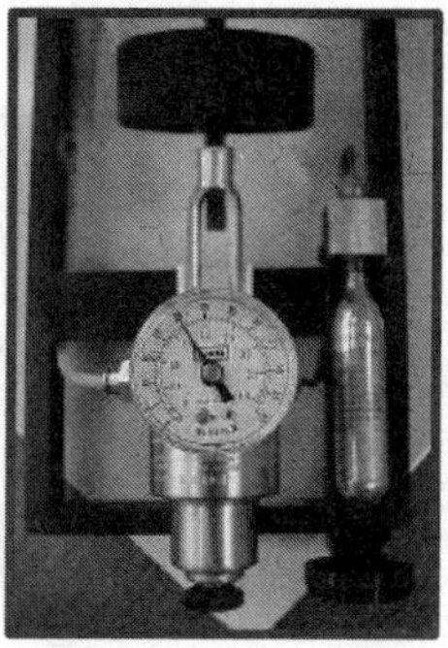

The English XL VIT was visually inspected before each testing session to ensure the security of fastenings, the alignment of the thrust cylinder, and the indicating pointer on the protractor.

Operating pressure of 25 PSI + or - 1.5 PSI was maintained for all tests.

Sanding was done according to the June 11, 1999 *Supplement to the XL Operations Manual.*

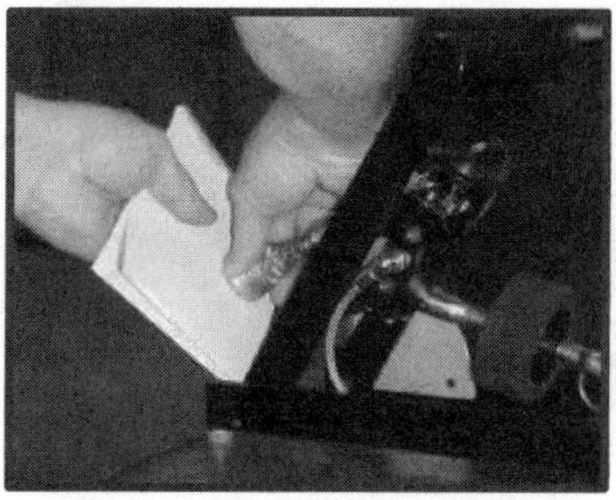

The Neolite test liner disk was sanded after each stroke that produced a slip. For wet testing, sanding was completed before each test session.

First, the XL was moved away from the tile (so that sanding dust would not fall onto the test zone).

The Neolite test liner disk was prepared by lightly sanding in a circulator motion for five cycles with180 grit silicon carbide sandpaper with a hard backing. Fresh sandpaper was used when the paper became visibly worn. The test foot was then brushed off and returned to the testing position. In addition to sanding, the disk was rotated about turn after each slip. The combination of sanding and rotation of the disk avoids the potential for polishing of the disk, which could affect test results.

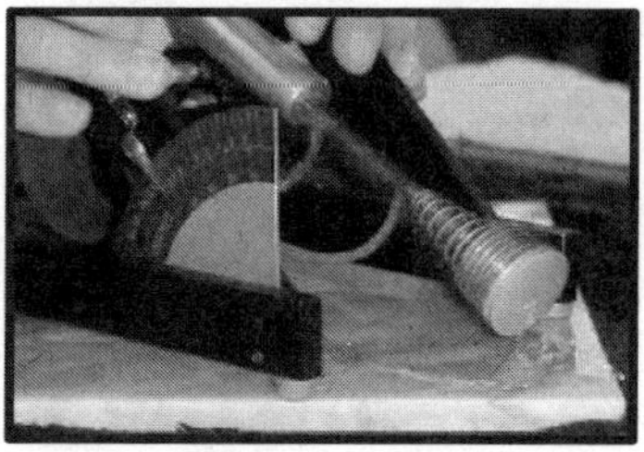

Wet Testing

Surfaces were first tested dry and then tested wet. Water was used for wet testing. Surfaces were wet in advance of actual testing to ensure that the surface material was adequately saturated. A thin, unbroken film of water was maintained on the surface.

Testing Process

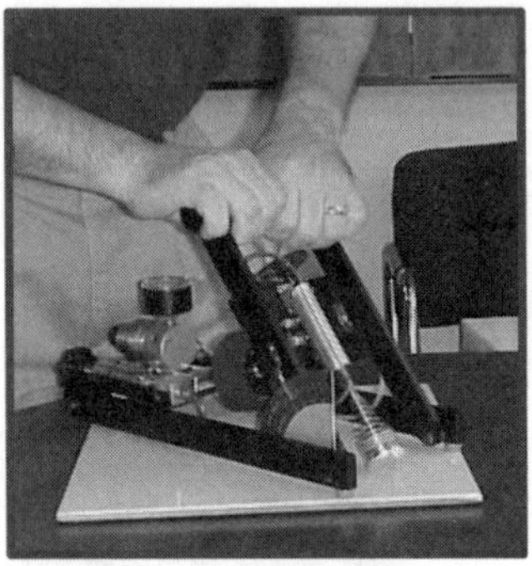

The starting point of the mast angle was estimated conservatively, to minimize the potential of an immediate slip. A relatively low slip index (a more vertical mast, such as 0.2 slip index reading) was used, gradually working up to higher slip index (more horizontal mast).

The hand wheel was turned about turn for each stroke. The actuating button was pressed for second and released.

The process was repeated until the first full-stroke slip occurred. The results were then read from the slip index protractor (rounded to the nearest 0.01), and documented using the attached spreadsheet.

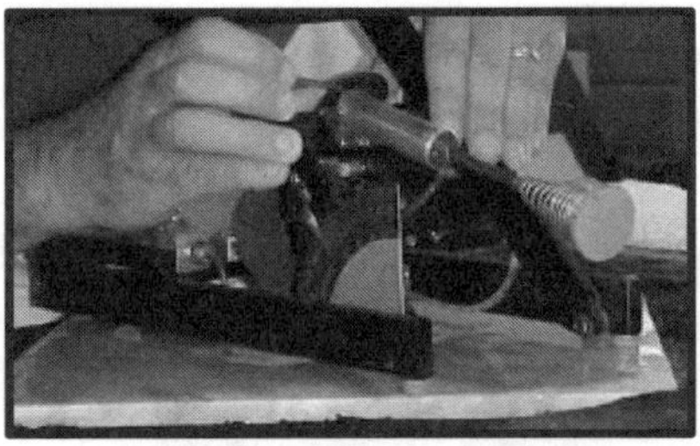

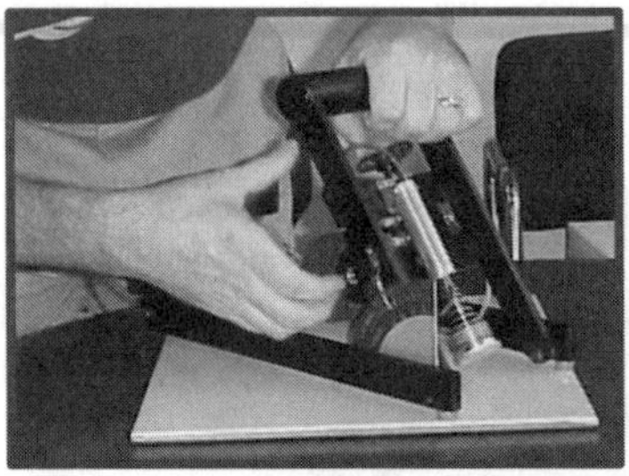

To ensure statistical reliability, three sets of four readings (one for each quadrant) were taken for each round of tests (e.g., readings on quadrants A, B, C, and D were taken three times for dry ceramic tile pretest).

ESIS Risk Control Services

Slip Resistant Treatment Study 2000

Exhibit: Statistical Analysis

Test Results by Group

The statistical analysis of test results was performed by David Underwood, Ph.D. A paired-comparison t-test was done, using the average from each set of four readings to obtain the probability of whether the numbers are the same. This probability ranges from 0 (no chance they are the same) to 1 (100% chance they are the same). Generally, if the probability is 0.05 or less, the numbers can be considered different. If a p value of 0.05 translates to 100*(1 - 05) = 95%, there is 95% confidence that the numbers are different.

Where the confidence factor is in the 95% range, the results of the testing are considered to be statistically sound and reliable.

Sample	P Value	Confidence
Group One		
Ceramic Dry	0.19	81%
Ceramic Wet	<0.001	+99%
Marble Dry	0.003	+99%
Marble Wet	<0.001	+99%
Group Two		
Ceramic Dry	<0.001	+99%
Ceramic Wet	<0.001	+99%
Marble Dry	<0.001	+99%
Marble Wet	<0.001	+99%
Group Three		
Ceramic Dry	0.02	98%
Ceramic Wet	0.004	+99%
Marble Dry	0.01	+99%
Marble Wet	0.148	85%
Group Four		
Ceramic Dry	0.001	+99%
Ceramic Wet	0.002	+99%
Marble Dry	0.10	90%
Marble Wet	0.006	+99%

Test Results by Group
(continued)

Sample	P Value	Confidence
Group Five		
Ceramic Dry	0.02	98%
Ceramic Wet	0.002	+99%
Marble Dry	0.34	66%
Marble Wet	0.53	47%
Group Six		
Ceramic Dry	0.01	99%
Ceramic Wet	<0.001	+99%
Marble Dry	N/A	N/A
Marble Wet	N/A	N/A
Group Seven		
Ceramic Dry	<0.001	+99%
Ceramic Wet	0.06	94%
Marble Dry	<0.001	+99%
Marble Wet	0.07	93%
Group Eight		
Ceramic Dry	0.02	98%
Ceramic Wet	0.13	87%
Marble Dry	0.52	48%
Marble Wet	0.03	97%
Group Nine		
Ceramic Dry	0.03	97%
Ceramic Wet	<0.001	+99%
Marble Dry	0.02	98%
Marble Wet	0.02	98%
Group Ten		
Ceramic Dry	0.04	96%
Ceramic Wet	0.02	98%
Marble Dry	<0.001	+99%
Marble Wet	0.06	94%

7 Footwear

7.1 INTRODUCTION

Falls are responsible for a significant portion of employee injuries. Aside from the obvious costs, employee injuries also interrupt customer service, and can affect profitability. Although it is unlikely that you will influence the general public, management can certainly exercise a much higher degree of control over the footwear worn by employees.

This chapter provides information on the elements of design and construction of slip resistant footwear, labeling and testing issues, advertising traps to avoid; general guidelines on selection of footwear in general; other protection features to consider; maintenance; and issues to consider when establishing a footwear policy. It also provides a brief overview of key international standards related to footwear slip resistance.

Clear and compelling evidence exists that using slip resistant footwear reduces accidents. In 2001, St. Lawrence University (Canton, NY) completed a pilot study by providing slip resistant footwear to its employees. The reduction in injury rates and workers' compensation claims of this small school resulted in savings of an estimated $100,000. Also, a food service operation employing 250 people at a major airport reduced slip and fall accidents to zero for over a year.

However, one make of footwear promoted as "slip resistant" may be significantly more or less slip resistant than another. Also, footwear that is slip resistant in one environment may not be in another. The effectiveness of slip resistant footwear depends not only on the efficacy of the design, but also the environmental conditions, type of floor surface and finish, and other factors. Beyond selection, maintenance and administration of footwear programs is needed in order to achieve success.

7.2 FOOTWEAR DESIGN FOR SLIP RESISTANCE

The types of footwear that employees are permitted to wear should be limited. In general, footwear with hard plastic or leather soles or heels should not be permitted, nor should soles with little or no tread pattern (e.g., smooth). Instead, footwear with slip resistant soles should be required.

7.2.1 Sole Compounds

The material of the heel and sole of footwear is a major factor in its performance as slip resistant (also see Chapter 4, Section 4.9, "Test Pad Material").

In general, softer compounds are more slip resistant than harder materials. For example, women's high-heeled shoes are often made from a very hard plastic, known as PVC (polyvinyl chloride). Even with a tread design, this material against a relatively smooth, hard walkway surface (such as marble, terrazzo, or ceramic) provides little slip resistance.

The consistency and life of materials should also be considered. Leather is an inconsistent material; its properties change over time, with wear, and when saturated with water, oil, or other such materials. As such, leather is a poor choice for footwear bottom material.

Some footwear bottom materials have a finite time in which they perform consistently. After that period, which could be as short as 12 months, the properties of the material change with wear and may not perform in the same way. Styrene-butadiene rubber (SBR), nitrile-butadiene rubber (NBR), and polyurethanes are some of the most commonly used footwear bottom materials. Similar to many other rubbers, they can be formulated in a wide range of hardness.

7.2.2 Tread Patterns

Tread patterns can significantly impact slip resistance performance, due to issues such as directionality, contaminant runoff, contact area, and impact of wear.

Tread patterns that run in the direction of travel are ill advised because they tend to accentuate rather than retard forward motion. Random patterns and patterns perpendicular to the direction of travel are more effective in providing slip resistance.

Patterns that produce enclosed areas are also not recommended. These areas can collect and trap water or other liquid contaminants. Having no path to disperse, the liquid is squeezed. If the liquid is unable to compress, hydroplaning can result (see Chapter 1).

Contact area is the percentage of the footwear bottom that makes contact with the walkway surface. In general, the greater the contact area, the better the slip resistance. At the same time, large unpatterned areas (especially the heel), while providing greater contact area, do not allow for liquid runoff, nor do they provide a means of gripping the surface.

7.2.3 General Guidelines for Shoe Design and Selection

Few published guidelines regarding shoe design and construction are available. The following are some recommendations published by SATRA Technology Centre, Ltd., U.K.:

Heel

- Round and patterned
- Square heel breast (acts as leading edge) as opposed to a rounded edge

Sole

- Flat, flexible bottom construction — Consider a low-density midsole that conforms to ground and maximizes contact area.
- Material that wears evenly and smoothly
- Consider wedge sole for indoor occupational footwear (e.g., catering, hospitals, sports footwear). This helps to provide the maximum contact area with the floor.

- A raised tread pattern extending over whole sole and heel area
- A pattern with leading edges in many directions (e.g., a cross hatch or similar design)

Cleat Patterns

- Cleat width between 3 to 20 mm
- Channel width at least 2 mm
- Well-defined square leading edges
- Radius internal corners (prevents sole cracking)
- Minimum depth of at least 2 mm

Slip resistant footwear bottom design guidelines are based on the SATRA Chart ("Slip Resistant Sole Design Diagram"), which is reproduced with the permission of SATRA (Figure 7.1). For more information, contact SATRA at http://www.satra.co.uk/.

7.3 LABELING

7.3.1 LABELING FOR USAGE

Although many factors may contribute to any injury, many injuries have a common contributing factor: improper footwear. Shoes are made with specific characteristics to provide the best attributes for a particular activity. For example, a sprinter's shoes are very lightweight, have almost no heel, and include a sturdy sole for flat-out speed. A linesman's boot has heavy, ankle-high leather uppers to prevent twisted ankles and a steel sole shank to ease pressures on the foot while standing on narrow telephone pole pegs.

Many specific attributes also create hazards for other types of activities. A tennis shoe provides good traction, but does not provide puncture resistance or toe protection.

So, the first step is to determine the activities performed and the types of contaminants prevalent in your facility, such as petroleum-based oils (auto oil, axle

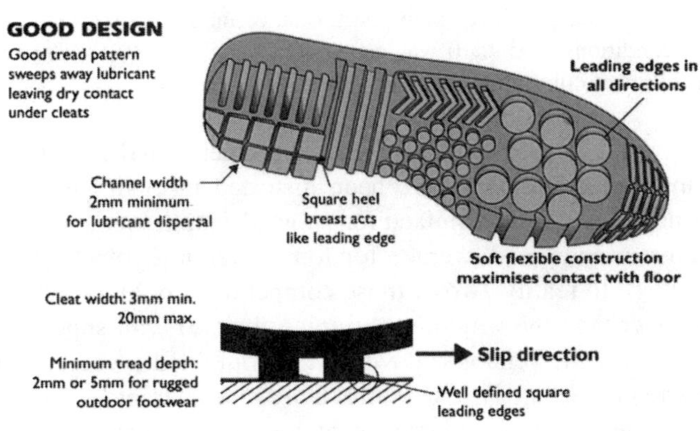

FIGURE 7.1 Attributes of "Good Sole Design" taken from SATRA slip resistance soling design guidelines.

grease, and/or lubricants), solvents/acids, or food-based oils (cooking oil, shortening, grease). Then, be sure the label indicates that the manufacturer recommends that particular type of footwear for such conditions.

7.3.2 Labeling for Slip Resistance Testing

Certain varieties of footwear on the market are promoted as "slip resistant." Although slip resistant footwear can be tested, most tests contemplate clean, dry floor surface conditions. Test method ASTM F489 (James Machine, see Chapter 4, Section 4.4) is the most commonly performed and cited test for footwear slip resistance, but it specifies dry testing only.

The SATRA TM 144 Whole Shoe Tester™ (see Chapter 8, Section 8.10.2) is preferred by many footwear industry professionals and is used extensively in Europe. The European Union is preparing to adopt such a method (see Section 7.10.1.3, "CEN"); however, independent studies regarding the efficacy of the method are not readily available. Some manufacturers of slip resistant footwear may also use ASTM F1677 and F1678 (see Chapter 4).

These methods do contemplate wet and contaminated conditions. One concern, however, is that only a portion of the shoe can be tested on these instruments. Thus, the overall performance of all the design aspects of the footwear cannot be engaged.

7.4 ADVERTISING

Caution must be exercised when evaluating product claims regarding the performance of slip resistant footwear. In some cases, vendors have cited wet or contaminated test results using a dry only test method (e.g., ASTM F489), which usually yields unrealistically higher results due to sticktion (Chapter 3, Section 3.7.2).

Self-serving slip resistance scales are sometimes used in an attempt to show superior performance of footwear products. In one example, one vendor indicated that:

> 0.35–0.50 was considered "acceptable" performance, and 0.50–0.60 was "good" for dry and wet conditions 0.05–0.10 was considered "fair," and 0.10–0.20 was "good" for oily and oily/wet conditions.

In addition, the vendor implied that these were government standards, but they were not.

In other instances, numbers have been distorted through improper averaging methods. In one example, a manufacturer showed results of 0.44 (oily) and 0.45 (oily/wet) against a combined average for four different competitors of 0.34 (oil) and 0.34 (oily/wet). In reality, two of those competitors could have had poor results (significantly lower than the vendor's), bringing the two with superior results (significantly higher than the vendor's) down to the combined average.

Other advertising methods use wording such as "restaurant tested and approved," which is too vague to be considered an endorsement. "Patent pending design," indicates only that the design may be the subject of a patent application, not that it is necessarily more effective than other designs.

7.5 OTHER SELECTION GUIDELINES

Comfort is an important factor in the selection of footwear. For the program to be successful, employees must actually wear the footwear. Footwear that is uncomfortable will make this less likely to happen, therefore:

- Employees should try on the footwear first.
- Their foot should be measured by the salesperson. If one foot is slightly larger than the other, the larger sized pair should be selected.
- If heavy socks or liners will be worn with the footwear, they should be worn while trying on the footwear before purchasing to ensure a proper fit.
- Because feet are the most swollen at the end of the day, employees should wait until then to shop for footwear.
- Footwear should not be selected on style. Comfort is more important.

7.6 OTHER PROTECTIVE FEATURES

In 1994, the Occupational Safety and Health Administration (OSHA) launched its first formal hazard assessment program, which required employers to institute personal protective equipment (PPE) programs. According to statistics from the Bureau of Labor Statistics (BLS), the result has been a reduction in foot and toe injuries range from 32 to 39%.

Depending on the environment in which the footwear is to be used, other protection features may also be needed. ANSI Z41-1999, *Personal Protection – Protective Footwear,* addresses most of these specifications, dealing primarily with foot armoring and control of electricity. OSHA 29 CFR Part 1910.136 references this document. Although these topics are beyond the scope of this chapter, additional protective features may include:

- Toe caps to guard against the impact of falling objects
- Puncture-resistant steel plated or other composite mid-soles to protect foot bottom from sharp objects
- Electric-shock-resistant footwear to insulate from electrical shock
- Static dissipative footwear to minimize the buildup of static electricity where sensitive equipment is present
- Conductive footwear for grounding when working with hazardous materials
- Metatarsal guards to protect the top of the foot from falling/rolling objects
- Ankle support for wet or sloping environments
- Anti-fatigue qualities, providing shock absorption, cushioning, and lightweight materials
- Thermal insulation to keep feet warm in cold temperatures
- Chemical resistance to protect from contact with certain caustic chemicals
- Water resistance in wet environments

7.7 MAINTENANCE

7.7.1 Keeping Clean

Inspection and maintenance is part of any effective program, and footwear is no different. Footwear should be checked for cleanliness and condition daily, prior to the start of work. The presence of liquid contaminants or solid matter wedged in tread patterns can reduce slip resistant properties. Disposable slip resistant shoe covers are available, but they are generally designed to last for one workday and should be discarded thereafter.

7.7.2 Wear/Replacement

Wear impacts the effectiveness of slip resistant footwear, but several factors influence the degree of wear. In any event, it is just a matter of time before slip resistance begins to deteriorate and the footwear needs to be replaced. The primary consideration is the effect of environmental and floor conditions on the footwear bottom material and tread pattern design. In general, walking on smooth surfaces tends to "polish" the footwear bottom, whereas walking on rougher surfaces tends to result in uneven wear or damage.

Upon inspection, signs of wear are usually clear: the rear of the heel is worn away and the sharp peaks of treads are shorter and flatter. Another consideration is simply the amount of use the footwear receives. In the absence of obvious signs of sudden damage, such as punctures, gouges, or cuts, some experts suggest that the life of average footwear is 6 months to 1 year.

7.8 FOOTWEAR PROGRAMS

7.8.1 Mandate or Recommend

Before instituting a slip resistant footwear program, it is important to seek legal counsel. Although a mandatory policy is likely to maximize footwear usage, it could also present potential legal exposures if improperly drafted or implemented. It may be helpful to request that footwear vendors provide sample footwear policies for you and your counsel to examine when designing your own footwear programs.

7.8.2 Purchase Options

It is advisable to review the legal and practical implementations of each option for footwear purchase. Issues such as labor and union agreements, the impact on employee morale, and record-keeping requirements need to be considered and balanced.

Purchase for Employees — It could be argued that slip resistant footwear, for the purposes of employee safety, is no different from any other type of personal protective equipment. In general, employees are not asked to purchase and maintain their own facemasks, hard hats, safety goggles, or respirators. Clearly, the downside of providing footwear for employees is the purchase price, but the benefits can certainly outweigh this consideration. Purchasing the footwear for your employees allows control over the kind of footwear worn. If consistency in look/style is important to your operations, this can also be specified. In addition, a purchase plan makes it easier to track the age and condition of footwear, permitting a system for scheduling replacing them in a timely fashion.

Employee Purchase — If employees are required to provide their own footwear, this should be clear at the time of hiring. The cost, along with criteria for acceptable footwear, should be provided in writing. It is often possible to negotiate discounts for employees to purchase selected types and styles of footwear through a specific vendor.

Payroll Deduction — Offering a voluntary payroll deduction option can make it easier for employees to purchase slip resistant footwear. The benefit is the ease with which footwear can be purchased, helping to make implementation more expedient. Provisions should be in place for handling reimbursement of costs when employees leave the company.

7.8.3 Enforcement

The policy should clearly state that any employee arriving at work in footwear other than that specified in the policy will be sent home. There should be a progressive disciplinary system to address repeated failure of employees to wear and maintain the specified footwear.

7.9 FEDERAL SPECIFICATION — USPS NO. 89C

USPS No. 89C is the *U.S. Postal Service Specification for Footwear.* A 1993 standard, this specification applies to the footwear worn by U.S. Postal Service employees. For slip resistance, it specifies the use of ASTM F489, *Static Coefficient of Friction of Shoe Sole and Heel Materials as Measured by the James Machine,* and requires a threshold of no less than 0.5. There is discussion that this standard soon may change.

7.10 INTERNATIONAL FOOTWEAR STANDARDS FOR SLIP RESISTANCE

Literally hundreds of domestic and international footwear-related standards are in existence. Although some slip resistance related specifications are contained within some general footwear standards, the following sections outline standards specific to footwear slip resistance. In most instances, the test apparatus of choice is the SATRA Whole Shoe Tester.

For information on U.S. Standards, see Chapter 4 (ASTM Standards Related to Pedestrian Safety). For details on each of the standard organizations mentioned next, see Chapter 8 (Overseas Slip Resistance Standards).

7.10.1 ISO

7.10.1.1 ISO/TR 11220: 1993

ISO/TR 11220: 1993 is the standard for *Footwear for Professional Use — Determination of Slip Resistance*. Placing the footwear on the testing surface with glycerin, applying a given load, and either moving the footwear horizontally in relation to the surface or moving the surface in relation to the footwear determines slip resistance. The frictional forces are measured and the dynamic coefficient of friction (DCOF) is calculated.

This standard is the responsibility of TC 94 (Foot Protection), for which BSI is the secretariat. It falls under SC 3 Work Group 1, *Determination of Slip Resistance,* which AFNOR is coordinating. It is still in the preliminary stages of work.

7.10.1.2 ISO/AWI 20878

ISO/AWI 20878 is the standard for *Footwear — Test Methods for Outsoles and Top Pieces — Slip Resistance*. This standard is the responsibility of TC 216 (Footwear), for which AFNOR is the secretariat. Still in the preparatory stage, its target date for publication is November 2003.

7.10.1.3 EUROPEAN (CEN)

7.10.1.3.1 PrEN 13287/PrEN 13287 rev

PrEN 13287/PrEN 13287 rev is the standard for *Safety, Protective and Occupational Footwear for Professional Use — Test Method for the Determination of Slip Resistance* (also see the British standards in Section 7.10.1.5). This standards falls under CEN/TC 161 (Foot and Leg Protectors), and is currently "Under Approval."

Although it is a generic method, the standard describes a protocol and instrument of considerable resemblance to the SATRA Whole Shoe Tester (PM144). It is expected that all CE-marked safety footwear will fall under this test method. The CE mark is the official marking required by the European Community for products sold in the European Community. It proves to the buyer — or user — that the product fulfills all essential safety and environmental requirements as they are defined in European Directives.

7.10.1.4 GERMAN — DIN 4843–100

DIN 4843–100 was published in August 1993, and it is available in German only. It is the standard for *Safety, Protective and Occupational Footwear; Slip Resistance, Metatarsal Protection, Protective Insert and Thermal Behaviour; Safety Requirements, Testing*.

7.10.1.5 BRITISH — DD 13287/EN 13287

This is a revision of an existing document, currently within the publication process. It is the responsibility of Committee PH/1, and publication is anticipated in June 2004, depending on the BSI project timeline. It is currently in the comment review stage.

8 Overseas Slip Resistance Standards

8.1 INTRODUCTION

Organizations with overseas facilities may find that U.S. standards related to pedestrian safety are not well recognized. Even the research community is somewhat segmented when performing this type of work. Whereas the U.S. has historically considered the static coefficient of friction (SCOF) as the most important measure related to pedestrian slip resistance, other countries have focused on the measurement of dynamic coefficient of friction (DCOF) as most representative measurement of slip resistance.

This chapter discusses the most commonly accepted slip resistance test methods overseas. An overview of the overseas standards-making organizations involved in slip resistance and their work in the field is also detailed. Finally, profiles of industry and other independent organizations involved in the study of slip resistance are presented.

8.2 SLIP AND FALL STATISTICS OVERSEAS

Perhaps not surprisingly, slip and fall accidents are one of the five leading causes of accidental death in other countries. According to the National Safety Council's International Accident Facts, falls are the number one (12 countries) or number two (20 countries) causes of death in 32 of the 37 countries that report such data. This is an average rank of 1.9, second only to motor vehicle accidents (a rank of 1.3). Countries with the highest number of fall deaths are:

- Germany (10,052) — Rank 1
- Italy (9624) — Rank 1
- France (9564) — Rank 1
- Poland (4805) — Rank 2
- Japan (4690) — Rank 2
- Mexico (4429) — Rank 2
- U.K. (4369) — Rank 1

With the exception of Russia and Mexico, the fall rates increase with age — mirroring the experience in the U.S.

Other statistics include:

- In the U.K., about 20% (or 40,000) of all occupational injuries are due to slips and falls (Manning, 1988; Thomas, 1991). Statistics from the U.K. indicate that 35% of all "non-fatal major" injuries and 21% of all "over-3-day" injuries are the result of falls on level surfaces. In high-risk industries, falls account for over 85% of worker accidents (Health & Safety Executive).
- In Germany, almost one in five work-related accidents are a result of slip and fall accidents, numbering almost a quarter million in 1997.
- In Australia, slips and falls resulted in 400,000 hospitalizations annually throughout the 1990s, 7000 deaths, and an estimated annual lifetime cost of $3.1 billion (see http://www.dbce.csiro.au/inno-web/0400/slips-falls.htm).

8.3 OVERSEAS STANDARD DEVELOPMENT

What about slipmeter methods in other countries? Could other researchers have developed and validated a method for wet testing that we could adopt in the U.S.?

Generally, U.S. standards for tribometers are the result of full consensus, requiring a "balanced" committee. In the case of ASTM international, no more than 50% of the committee can be producers of related products, and committee representation must be from a wide range of interests, including footwear, flooring, steel, consultants, and the general public. This is known as balancing a committee, intended so that no single interest group is able to exert undue influence in how a standard is developed or its requirements. In addition, there is a thorough appeal process for members with objections to the fairness of the development process of the standard. NFPA International (formerly the National Fire Protection Association) has similar processes. The full consensus approach is intended to arrive at viable standards that provide protection to the public while being reasonable enough to be implemented by industry.

Overseas, few organizations develop standards by the U.S. definition of full consensus. They may be funded, written, and published primarily by commercial groups with a vested financial interest in industry-friendly standards. Although these organizations may ostensibly welcome the participation of all parties, there is no requirement to maintain a specific balance of interests. In many committees, the end users (consumers) are poorly represented. Without balance, there is an understandably lower level of credibility and acceptance of resulting standards.

Although not seen as an issue overseas, safety professionals in the U.S. would consider such practices to produce biased standards. Therefore, from the perspective of the U.S., overseas standards developed primarily by vested interests must be approached cautiously. None of the following test methods discussed in this chapter (e.g., ramp test, pendulum, tortus et al.) has U.S. standards of any kind.

Another critical difference between ASTM standards and overseas standards has to do with validation of the test method. Whereas ASTM test methods require interlaboratory studies and the development of research reports to document the degree of accuracy, repeatability, and reproducibility of the test method, few overseas standards-making organizations have such requirements. Essentially, ASTM requires proof that the method works as intended through a process of testing and study under real world conditions. However, many overseas test methods are issued and widely used even though their viability remains unproven.

Note: The following information on standards activities must be read as a snapshot in time. Standards are in continual updating and development. It is recommended that the reader consult the Web links provided to determine the status of standards activities and obtain the current edition of standards cited herein.

8.4 RAMP TESTS

Ramp tests originated in Germany (see Figure 8.1), and have been adopted by the Australia/New Zealand cooperative. DIN 51097 and DIN 51130 require test persons to walk on various wet tiles. The angle of the ramp is gradually increased until the person begins to slip.

An interesting feature of these standards is the use of a classification system to provide guidance selecting materials with the appropriate level of slip resistance for a given area, based primarily on the activities performed and the contaminants present or likely to be present.

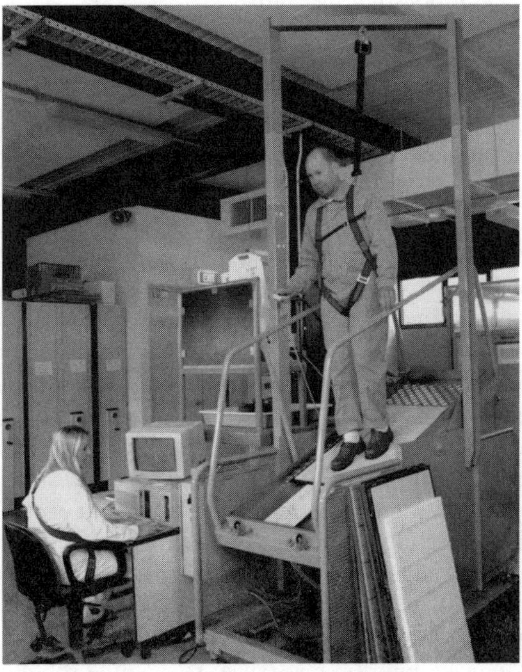

FIGURE 8.1 A German ramp test in process. Photograph courtesy of CSIRO.

At first glance, this approach makes some sense. Instead of using a device as a surrogate for walking, why not use people? After all, if we are concerned with people slipping and falling, we should just go to the source.

Perhaps, but the ramp test approach has some issues. Experts agree that a person's awareness of a potentially slippery surface can influence the way he or she traverses that area. If you see the ice or water, you will adjust your gait accordingly, and probably cross it without incident. It is when you are unaware of the hazard and expect the same level of traction that you have had that slips are most likely to occur. Let us now look at ramp tests:

- People selected to participate in a ramp test expect a slippery surface. No amount of preparation or instruction will change that. It likely they will alter their gait in anticipation of a slippery surface. As a result, they will perform much better on a ramp test than they would when encountering an unexpectedly slippery surface in real life. K. Schuster from BIA (see Section 8.10.6) concluded that tests with human subjects under such conditions are irrelevant because they essentially eliminate the element of surprise.
- As is known by many researchers in biomechanics, people walk differently on an incline than on a level surface. Slipping at a certain point on an incline cannot be correlated to slipping on the same surface were it level. Because the biomechanical factors of human ambulation are so vastly different in such situations, this test method should not purport to be valid for a condition it does not measure.
- People are different, and the length, speed, and biases in their gaits vary. Those factors also change with age. Generally, ramp tests have involved only younger, able-bodied individuals, hardly representative of the population at large. Although tribometers provide a consistent means of measurement by limiting variables to the surface being tested, it is difficult to argue that ramp tests do so.
- The test method specifies the use of as few as two test subjects, a statistically inadequate sample hardly sufficient to provide a basis for validating the results. The two subjects selected could easily be anomalous, thus delivering measurements that bear no resemblance to actual conditions.
- Ramp tests refer to "standard test shoes." This is still another variable that must be accounted for. In fact, the German DIN committee has been faced with the inability to obtain the specified type and quality of Bottrop footwear needed for the test.
- Another barrier to the use of this as a reasonable test standard is the cost. The construction of ramp facilities and the use of test people plus operators make it cost prohibitive to most. The calibration board tiles alone run almost $7000. In addition, at present, the reserve stock of these tiles is almost used up.
- In some instances, pretesting of tiles with an alternate method (e.g., pendulum) indicate low slip resistance. During the subsequent ramp test, these suspect tiles are deliberately placed at the bottom of the ramp to

ensure they are not being stood on at the start of each walk down the ramp. This can result in inappropriately optimistic test results.

In essence, ramp tests involve many biases and variables, bringing into question whether they can be considered a viable method for evaluating the traction of level walkway surfaces. This being the case, reasonable efforts should be made to minimize those variables. Part of that effort should include well-designed and conducted ruggedness testing and an interlaboratory study. Because of the numerous and complex variables involved, and the ease with which the results could be manipulated, such studies are fundamental to the validating this test method.

8.5 PENDULUM TESTERS

The original pendulum tester, the Sigler, was developed by Percy Sigler at the U.S. National Bureau of Standards (NBS) in the 1940s and dubbed the "NBS Standard Dynamic COF Tester." Since then, the Sigler has fallen out of U.S. standards for pedestrian slip resistance (there was, at one time, a federal and an NBS standard for this device), due to the inability to correlate the results of the instrument with human perception of slipperiness. In the 1950s, ASTM D21 on Polishes studied the Sigler and the James Machine as potential test methods for slip resistance. However, only a James Machine standard (in the form of test method D2047) was ever developed and published (see Figure 8.2).

The pendulum is based on the Izod principle. A pendulum rotates on a spindle attached to a vertical pillar. The end of the pendulum arm holds a foot fitted with a (usually rubber) material ranging from 1.25 to 3 in. The pendulum is released from the horizontal position so that it strikes the test foot under a constant velocity. The distance the test foot travels after striking the surface determines the friction of the floor surface, which is read from the scale.

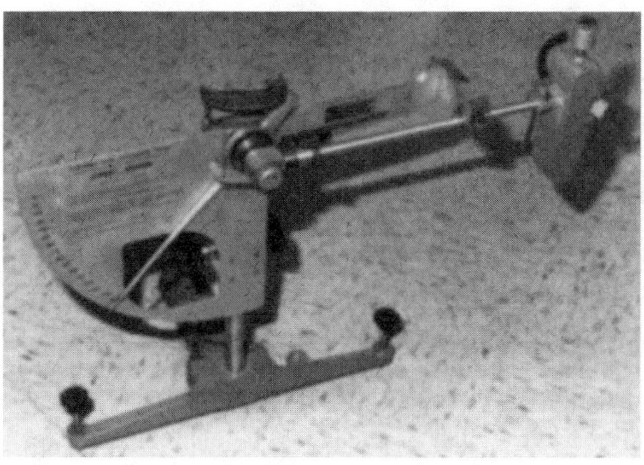

FIGURE 8.2 A Stanley pendulum tester, quite similar to the British portable skid tester (BPST). Photograph courtesy of CSIRO.

TABLE 8.1
Greater London Council Pendulum Thresholds

Original GLC Guideline (TRRL Test Foot)		Guideline as modified by James (4S Test Foot)	
Pendulum Reading	**Interpretation**	**Pendulum Reading**	**Interpretation**
75 and above	Excellent	65 and above	Very good
40 to 74	Satisfactory	35 to 64	Good
20 to 39	Marginal	25 to 34	Marginal
19 and below	Dangerous	24 and below	Unsatisfactory

The pendulum provides readers between 0 and 150, often referred to as pendulum numbers. Because pendulum numbers are unique and thus difficult to correlate with other measurements, guidelines by the Greater London Council can be used to interpret test results (Table 8.1). A subsequent variation of the Sigler, the TRRL Tester (and known in the U.S. as the British Portable Skid Tester or BPST) does have an ASTM standard, but not for pedestrian slip resistance. ASTM E-303, Method for Measuring Surface Frictional Properties using the British Pendulum Tester, is approved for the evaluation of the skid resistance of roadways for vehicular use. The term "skid-resistance" is defined to correlate the performance of a vehicle with patterned tires braking with locked wheels on a wet road at 50 km/h (30 mph). The BPST was developed a British government organization, Road Research Laboratory (or Transport Research Laboratory). For more information on the BPST, see http://www.munro-group.co.uk/skid.htm and http://www.wessexengineering.co.uk/product5.asp. In the U.K., the BPST was used for evaluating pedestrian slip resistance, despite the fact that at eight miles per hour (about 200 times faster than the movement of the Tortus test foot), the slider speed is much greater than that of a person's heel striking the floor during walking.

Practical problems with this device for measuring pedestrian slip resistance include the dynamics and operation of pendulum devices in general. Of particular concern is the excessive velocity at which the machine operates, bearing no relation to that of human ambulation. Research conducted in the 1970s by ASTM F15.03 (Consumer Safety) determined that the pendulum devices showed significant variation across the test surface, making a reasonable correlation of these results to a single slip resistance value impractical. The same conclusion was reached in the Bucknell ASTM workshop in 1991, and in a separate research project by the NBS in the late 1970s (in which NBS concluded that it would be difficult, if not impossible, to relate friction directly to the energy loss).

Although it is known that slip resistance increases with surface roughness, a study RAPRA (see Section 8.10.1) of the pendulum concluded that there is a poor correlation between wet friction as measured by this instrument and surface roughness. Likewise, pendulum instruments are unable to accurately meter surfaces that slope by more than 5°, or surfaces that have irregular profiles (e.g., non-smooth surfaces).

Still another issue is usability. Because the device is complex and difficult to operate, the results are highly subject to operator error. A full interlaboratory study by Transit New Zealand, which examined repeatability and reproducibility, indicated that operator practice can have a significant influence on results. The range of results for repeatability was found to be moderate to large (ranging from 4 to 25 pendulum numbers) and the range for reproducibility was always large (at 20 to 34 pendulum numbers).

There is a high dependency on the degree of slope as well as the direction of travel (up or down). Measuring up a slope of 15% yields results 30 to 50% higher than level surface measurements. Measuring down a similar slope yields results 20 to 30% lower than those on level surfaces (Dravitzki and Potter, 1997).

Finally, the calculation and interpretation of its readings is intricate, requiring the insertion of three values into an algebraic formula. In fact, in the NBS Preliminary Study of the Slipperiness of Flooring (NBSIR 74-613), the results of the BPST had to be expressed in "British Portable Skid Tester Numbers" because they are not readily convertible to coefficient of friction numbers. The external calibration requirements for this complex instrument allow up to 2 years between calibrations.

Understandably, the pendulum tester is not suitable for assessing the slip resistance of resilient flooring materials. Because it relies upon a loss of energy to obtain a measurement of slip resistance, and a resilient surface tends to absorb energy, inaccurate results can be expected. The tendency of resilient materials to deform under the force of the pendulum may also contribute to the lower readings obtained from these materials.

The pendulum tester (particularly the BPST) was selected for European (and therefore international) standardization purely by a process of elimination. A field test method for wet measurement was needed, and the preferred overseas technologies were not viable. The ramp test is a laboratory apparatus, and the Tortus was acknowledged to be unsuitable for wet testing, leaving only the pendulum.

8.6 DIGITIZED DRAGSLEDS

Originally developed in 1980 by British Ceramic Research Association (Ceram) as a bench test for ceramic floor tiles, the original patent for the Tortus has expired, and there are several look-alikes commercially available. The Tortus II (British), Sellmaier (German), FFT (Floor Friction Tester), Gabbrielli (Italian), and FSC2000 are variations of the same technology.

The Tortus and its successors are four wheeled, self-propelled, electronic devices based on dragsled principles. Test pad material varies (the Tortus II uses 4S rubber while the Sellmaier uses several different materials). As the test pad is dragged across the floor, it records frictional forces and displays and prints the values. Mean values are estimated from this data. The drag on the 4.5 mm circular disc is measured through leaf springs. The original Tortus required an electrical connection, but subsequent versions are battery-powered. The contact area and load was intended to reproduce the area and pressure of a heel striking the ground. However, the movement of the Tortus test foot along the floor is quite unlike human ambulation in that it is dragged in continuous contact with the walkway surface.

Forceplate data from the 1991 Bucknell workshop conducted by ASTM F13 (in which several other tribometers were also evaluated) demonstrates the erratic and unstable output of this class of tester, and which produces results similar to the variable

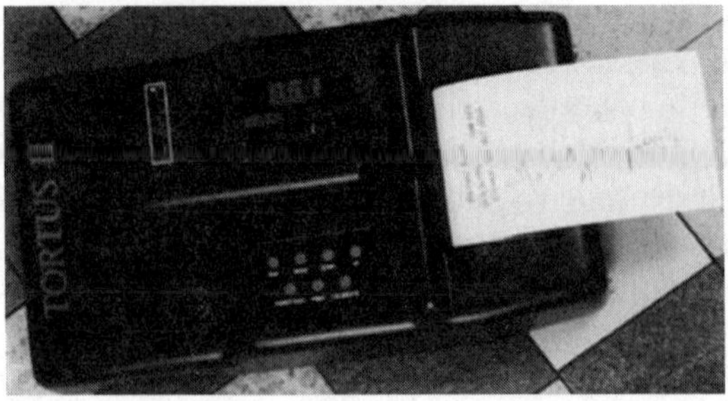

FIGURE 8.3 A subsequent incarnation of the original, the Tortus II, is powered by an internal battery. Photograph courtesy of CSIRO.

results of Horizontal Pull Slip Meter, another dragsled device, when performing wet testing. This was revealed by forceplate analysis because the instrument has a built-in filter that averages needle indications to make them appear less erratic. This averaging of greatly fluctuating readings leads to inconsistent and questionable results.

A British study likewise reported that this instrument tends to overestimate slip resistance due to the high traction properties of the standard slider, and its inability to account for hydroplaning on wet surfaces. In addition, an Australian study found high variability between the test results of different operators (Bowman, 1992). And like the pendulum, the Tortus is also incapable of accurately measuring surfaces that slope in excess of 5°, or non-smooth surfaces.

Even under dry conditions, the precision of the Tortus is questionable. A paper presented in 1997 by a distributor of the Tortus, provides the results of a dry test round robin involving 12 machines, one-third of which were done at the same laboratory (Martin and Dimopoulos, 1997). Even so, the results demonstrated poor precision (see Table 8.4).

The paper goes on to state that "It is difficult to explain these fluctuations other than to attribute them to tile preparation …" (see Figure 8.3). This device has several disadvantages. Major issues include:

- As a dragsled class of tribometer, the instrument in no way emulates human ambulation, so its readings are not meaningfully related to the human perception of walking.
- Because the instrument is considered to be simulating the action of a pedestrian moving cautiously across a floor, this becomes a test of greatly limited benefit.
- In a study of the Tortus at the ASTM F13 Bucknell workshop in 1991, readings from this instrument were the result of a series of stick-slip events caused by the foot sticking then jumping and sticking again — continuously. The actual readout is some average between the force build-up before the foot jumps (very high slip resistance) and the drift while it moves to a location where it remains stationary (very low slip resistance).
- Significant anomalies in readings occur in that readings often do not match subjective option. In one example, the Tortus delivers very high readings on very smooth surfaces. Surfaces that are patterned with raised pyramid,

stud, or rib designs, and those with large grit deliver unexpectedly low slip resistance readings. It is theorized that the reason for some of these anomalies is that the small size (and configuration) of the test foot at such a slow pace allows it to travel "over and down the profile without measuring its true effect in providing a slip resistant surface." (Dravitzki and Potter, 1997).

- The Tortus is not reliable for wet testing, due in part to the lack of adequate wheel traction, and the problem of sticktion. Even the new AS/NZ 4586 standard (*Slip Resistance Classification of New Pedestrian Surface Materials*) does not list this device for wet testing. This has been shown as an adhesion (or sticktion) problem developing between the test foot and the walkway surface due to the time delay between the application of horizontal and vertical forces (Bowman, 1992). In addition, studies have demonstrated poor correlation with subjective assessment of slip resistance. In these studies, the Tortus readings on virtually all wet surfaces were in the dangerous range (Strandberg, 1985; Harris and Shaw, 1988; Proctor and Coleman, 1988). A study by RAPRA (see Section 8.10.1) resulted in the conclusion that "the Tortus instrument is not at all reliable in wet conditions."
- There is no U.S. standard recognizing this class of tribometer as a valid test device, nor are there plans to develop one.
- The appropriateness of the test pad is questionable because, unlike heels, they are convex or cylindrical. It has been noted that the test foot contacts the floor not flatly, but at one edge. The walkway surface would need to be perfectly plane for flat contact to be made and maintained with the low pressure applied.

Although the original Tortus is no longer manufactured, more information about the Tortus II, developed by Severen Science based on earlier Tortus floor friction testers, can be found at http://www.severnscience.co.uk/pages/tortus.html and Mastrad at http://www.mastrad.com/tortus.htm.

8.7 OTHER DRAGSLEDS

As in the U.S., a variety of other dragsled-class instruments are used overseas, few of which have gained prominence. Among them are:

- The *Schuster Machine* (Germany) is quite similar to the ASTM C1028 (see Chapter 4), in that it is a manually pulled sledge manual, although the dynamometer is built-in.
- The *Hoechst Device* is more like an HPS (ASTM F609), a mechanically driven instrument, with three small circular test feet (chromium plated). It is also of German manufacture.
- The *CEBTP Skidmeter* consists of a block of tire rubber pulled by along two cylindrical rails by an electrically braked motor and a reduction gearbox. Developed in France by the Centre Experimental de Recherches et d'Etudes du Batiment et des TRAVAUX Publics (CEBTP), this presumably portable device consists of a substantial amount of equipment to operate.

As with any tribometer of this class, these dragsleds are unsuitable for wet testing due to "stick-slip" (see Chapters 3 and 4), and even under dry conditions they do not in any way relate to the mechanics of human ambulation. Although Germany has a DIN standard for a dragsled meter, none of these instruments are being considered for CEN or ISO standards at this time.

8.8 PORTABLE FRICTION TESTER

Developed by the Swedish National Road and Transport Research Institute, the PFT (Figure 8.4), or portable friction tester was originally designed to measure the friction on road markings (see http://www.tft.lth.se/kfbkonf/5bergstromnew.PDF). Its use was later expanded to include the friction on bicycle paths, and finally expanded even further to use for measuring pedestrian slip resistance. It has been referred to as a braked-wheel/skiddometer instrument in which there is an axel torque from braked rolling wheel.

Also known as FIDO, this instrument was found to be highly operator-dependent, particularly with regard to maintaining a constant horizontal velocity. It is clear that the friction model has little to do with human locomotion, yet it is still used by some overseas for pedestrian safety studies and floor slip resistance evaluation. The Finnish Institute of Occupational Health (FIOH) recently based a prototype tribometer on the same principles as FIDO in which six test pads are mounted on a pneumatic wheel driven by a DC motor. There is no U.S. standard, nor is one even being considered. In fact, there is no known overseas standard either.

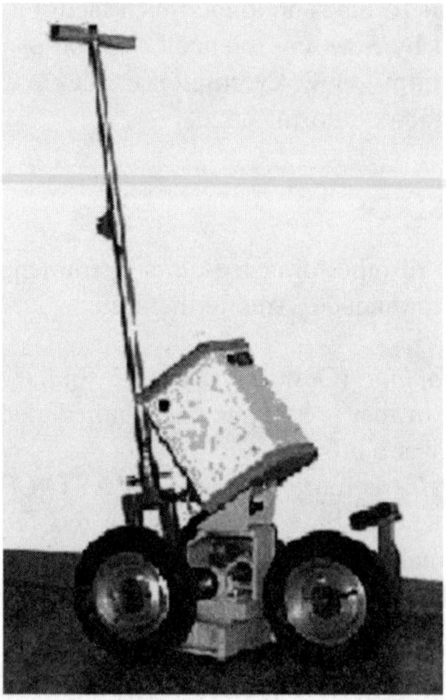

FIGURE 8.4 The Swedish portable friction tester (PFT or FIDO).

8.9 INTERNATIONAL STANDARDS

The standards that follow primarily deal with measurement and assessment of slip resistance of walkway surfaces, or are referenced by such standards. Footwear related slip resistance standards are also numerous, and are not the focus of this section.

Three primary sources of information are available about access to international standards, regulations, and related documents. Each source can be searched by document number, title, or key words:

- **Global Engineering Documents (GED)** at http://global.Ihs.com — Established in 1959, GED serves as a comprehensive source of technical industry standards and government and military standards. Most documents are available for download in Adobe Acrobat (PDF) format.
- **NSSN: A National Resource for Global Standards** at http://www.nssn.org — This is a comprehensive data network on developing and approved national, foreign, regional and international standards and regulatory documents. NSSN standards are products of the American National Standards Institute (ANSI). Part of NSSN is the STAR Service (Standards Tracking and Alerting Service), which allow users to establish profiles and track development standards.
- **ANSI Electronic Standards Store** at http://webstore.ansi.org/anisdocstore/default.asp

8.9.1 European Standards

In Europe, the ramp and pendulum test methods for measuring slip resistance have a strong following; however, the European Union is far from a consensus. Some countries prefer a Tortus-style instrument, and others are promoting standards for dragsled devices. Consensus on this issue in the EU does not appear to be achievable in the near future (see http://www.cenorm.be).

8.9.1.1 About CEN

European standards related to slip resistance are developed by a variety of different committees of CEN (Comite Europeen de Normalisation), the European Committee for Standardization. Following is a list of committees and slip resistance standards in process.

CEN's mission is to promote voluntary technical harmonization in Europe in conjunction with worldwide bodies and its partners in Europe. Many see this as an initiative to protect European industry from foreign incursions. The National Members are the "only effective" Members according to Belgian law under which CEN is registered as a nonprofit, international scientific and technical organization. Members are the national standards bodies of the EU and European Fair Trade Association (EFTA) countries and the Czech Republic.

8.9.1.2 CEN Standards Process

The members develop and vote for the ratification of European Standards. They must implement such standards as national standards, withdrawing all conflicting national standards on the same subject. In time, all European countries are expected to have CEN standards in place.

Through the Vienna Agreement, CEN and ISO have agreed to jointly develop standards. Once developed, CEN standards will almost certainly also become ISO standards. For more information on the relationship of CEN with ISO, see Section 8.9.8.

ANSI is the U.S. representative to CEN. As a nonmember nation, ANSI does not have a vote. Having a vote would obligate the U.S. to implement CEN standards and withdraw comparable U.S. standards, just as CEN member nations are required to.

The process begins with the establishment of a technical committee and project slate of standards. Draft standards are developed or adapted from one of the member countries. Next, each country's designated voting entity within CEN (for example, DIN represents Germany) ballots the draft in their own country. The technical committee then meets to finalize the document.

The designation "EN" signifies that the document is an approved standard that has been implemented by member countries. The designation "ENV" is a European Pre-standard, which is a prospective or provisional standard. ENVs are used when accelerated standards development is needed due to high rates of innovation (e.g., computer technology) or when there is an immediate need for the information. The designation "prEN" signifies a draft document that has not yet been approved or implemented.

8.9.1.3 CEN Slip Resistance Standards and Drafts

It appears as though separate CEN standards will be used for different materials (e.g., a ceramics method, a laminate method), long before unification into a single set of standards. BSI (British Standards Institute) estimates that it will take until around 2011 before these standards are harmonized.

8.9.1.3.1 CEN/TC 134

CEN/TC 134 is the standard for resilient textile and laminate floor coverings (see http://www.cenorm.be/standardization/tech_bodies/cen_bp/workpro/tc134.htm). *PrEN 13893 — (Draft) Resilient, Laminate and Textile Floor Coverings — Parameters for the Measurement of Dynamic Coefficient of Friction on Floor Surfaces.*

This document outlines the protocol for obtaining DCOF readings, but does not specify a test instrument. Rather it is designed to be a framework for any DCOF instrument (e.g., pendulum), specifying a leather test pad prepared with 320-grit sandpaper. It is important to note that the scope of this standard is limited to dry testing only.

This standard is currently "Under Approval," meaning that it is an active work item at a stage between the beginning of the inquiry and the end of a formal vote. In other words, it has been developed, but has not yet been approved. It is primarily a product of the British Standards Institute (BSI), which also acts as the secretariat of this technical committee.

The document *PrEN 13845 — (Draft) Resilient Floor Coverings — Polyvinyl Chloride Floor Coverings with Enhanced Slip Resistance — Specification* is also now "Under Approval."

8.9.1.3.2 CEN/TC 246

CEN/TC 246 is the standard for natural stones (see http://www.cenorm.be/standardization/tech_bodies/cen_bp/workpro/tc246.htm), *PrEN 14231 – (Draft) Natural Stones Test Methods – Determination of Slip Resistance by Means of the Pendulum Tester.* This document is also now "Under Approval."

8.9.1.3.3 CEN/TC 67

CEN/TC 67 is the standard for ceramic tiles (see http://www.cenorm.be/standardization/tech_bodies/cen_bp/workpro/tc067.htm), *PrEN 13552 (Draft) Ceramic Tiles – Determination of Coefficient of Friction.*

Based on an earlier draft of this document, this standard specifies the use of any of several test instruments, including the dynamic slider (e.g., Tortus), static slider (e.g., C1028), inclined platform (e.g., ramp test), pendulum (e.g., BPST). Except for the inclined platform, all are permitted for field testing in dry or wet conditions. It specifies a 4S rubber test foot prepared with 400-grit sandpaper. The inclined platform is essentially the DIN oil-coated ramp method, a laboratory test that must be done with 10W30 engine oil.

This document is also now "Under Approval." Attempts have been made to pass this standard for several years without success, due in large part to disagreement between member countries regarding the appropriateness of one test method or another.

8.9.2 German Standards

According to German regulations (see http://www.en.din.de), walkways must be slip resistant to comply with the Workplace Order and the Accident Prevention Regulation "General Regulations" (VBG 1). Standards in Germany are promulgated by the Deutsches Institut fur Normung e.V., also known as DIN. DIN, the German Institute for Standardization, is a registered association, founded in 1917. Its head office is in Berlin. Since 1975, it has been recognized by the German government as the national standards body and represents German interests at international and European level.

External experts, numbering 26,000, carry out standards work by serve as voluntary delegates in more than 4000 committees. Draft standards are published for public comment, and all comments are reviewed before final publication of the standard. Published standards are reviewed for continuing relevance every 5 years, at least.

Standards related to slip resistance are developed in Working Group NMP 882 "Tests on the Slip Resistance of Floor Coverings" of the Normenausschuss Materialprufung (materials testing standards committee).

8.9.2.1 DIN 18032 P2

DIN 18032 P2, with a publication date of February 1996 and available in German only, is the standard for *Sport Halls; Halls for Gymnastics and Games; Floors for Sporting Activities; Requirements, Testing.*

This standard specifies the use of the Stuttgart-Tester (or SST) for the measurement of friction. Originally developed in the 1960s, this semiportable instrument consists of a vertical shaft supported by a frame. The shaft moves downward when turned clockwise and upward when turned counterclockwise. A test foot is mounted on a pivot to the base of the shaft. A constant torque is applied by a steel wire wound over a winding drum and down onto the shaft. The wire runs over a guide pulley and is tensioned by a freely suspended 5-kg weight, which drives the shaft. The test foot is equipped with a strain gauge or piezo-electric device for measuring torque. The test foot surface consists of three skids that are 20 mm wide and 45 mm long, of a 50 mm diameter cylinder, and surfaced with leather. To operate, the shaft is raised (causing the steel wire to wind onto the drum) and is released so that the weights drive the shaft downward. The test foot contacts the surface, and the rotation of the shaft is breaked by the friction, measured as torque. There is no known manufacturer of the instrument.

8.9.2.2 DIN 51 097

DIN 51 097, with a publication date of November 1992, is the standard for *Testing of Floor Coverings; Determination of the Anti-Slip Properties; Wet-Loaded Barefoot Areas; Walking Method; Ramp Test.*

This standard is intended to provide a means to measure floor-covering materials intended for use in areas which are normally wet and walked upon barefoot (e.g., hospitals, changing rooms, washrooms, showers, swimming pools). It calls for a minimum of two subjects to walk on a gradually increasing inclined plane barefoot on a wet ramp. The results are rated in Table 8.2.

8.9.2.3 DIN 51 130

DIN 51 130, with a publication date of November 1992 and available in German only, is the standard for *Testing of Floor Coverings; Determination of the Anti-Slip Properties; Workrooms and Fields of Activities with Raised Slip Danger; Walking Method; Ramp Test.*

This standard is intended to provide a means to measure floor-covering materials intended for use in workrooms and public areas. It calls for a minimum of two subjects to walk on a gradually increasing inclined plane with specific footwear on an oil-coated ramp. The results are rated in Table 8.3.

8.9.2.4 DIN 51 131

DIN 51 131, with a publication date of July 1999 and available in German only, is the standard for *Testing of Floor Coverings — Determination of the Anti-Slip*

TABLE 8.2
DIN 51 097 Valuation Groups

Valuation Group	Angle of Inclination
A	> 12 degrees
B	> 18 degrees
C	> 24 degrees

TABLE 8.3
DIN 51 130 Valuation Groups

Valuation Group	Angle of Inclination	Rating
R9	> 3–10 degrees	Low static friction
R10	> 10–19 degrees	Normal static friction
R11	> 19–27 degrees	Increased static friction
R12	> 27–35 degrees	High static friction
R13	> 35 degrees	Very high static friction

TABLE 8.4
Tortus Round Robin (Dry)

Tile	High Reading	Low Reading	Average	SD
A (Smooth)	.86	.44	.66	.11
B (Textured)	.94	.70	.87	.06
C (Textured)	.78	.63	.71	.05

Properties — Measurement of Sliding Friction Coefficient. This test method specifies the use of a dragsled class of tribometer.

8.9.3 British Standards

British standards are the responsibility of BSI (http://www.bsi-global.com/group.xalter), the British Standards Institute. Formed in 1901 under a royal Charter, BSI was created to help British industry compete in European and international trade markets. The BSI Group began life as a committee of engineers determined to standardize the number and type of steel sections. Currently, BSI operates in 112 countries and represents the U.K. for European and international standardization.

British standard BS 0 specifies how BS committees are to set up and operate. British standards are subject to public comment before being published, although drafts must be purchased for review. Although other committees also develop pedestrian slip related standards, Committee B/556 is the primary committee for pedestrian slip measurement and is represented by manufacturers, building/materials research organizations, testing laboratories, the Health & Safety Executive (HSE), architects/consulting engineers, and certifying organizations; Committee B/556 is said to be well balanced.

8.9.3.1 Committee B/556

Committee B/556 coordinates pedestrian slip resistance for standard *BS 7976-1 Pendulum Testers — The Pendulum Tester Part 1: Specification.*

This standard describes the use and calibration of the pendulum tester, providing a detailed protocol for testing and an on-site validation procedure in which the user can confirm that the test is being performed correctly and that the instrument is set up and operating properly. Now in the comment review phase of the standards process, publication is anticipated in January 2003.

8.9.3.2 Committee B/208

Committee B/208 oversees stairs and walkways for standard *BS 5395, Part 1 Stairs, Ladders & Walkways. Code of Practice for the Design, Construction and Maintenance of Straight Stairs and Winders, which was published in June 2000.*

This standard refers to the BPST (British Portable Skid Tester), a pendulum class tribometer as apparatus to measure the slip resistance of walkway surfaces. Guideline thresholds are as follows:

> 0.75 Good (Suitable for “high risk” areas)
0.40 – 0.75 Adequate (Suitable for “normal use”)
0.20 – 0.39 Poor, May Be Unsafe
< 0.20 Very Poor, Unsafe

8.9.3.3 Committee B/545

Committee B/545 oversees natural stone; it is responsible for BS EN 14231, (CEN standard PrEN 14231). The project is in the publication process, was ratified in 2003.

8.9.3.4 Committee B/539

Committee B/539 oversees ceramic tiles and other rigid tiling. This committee ballots CEN draft standards relating to ceramic tiles. It is currently balloting 99/109274 DC (CEN standard PrEN 13552 1999).

8.9.3.5 Committee PRI/60

This committee ballots CEN draft standards relating to resilient floor coverings. They are currently balloting 00/120903 DC (CEN standard PrEN 13845 2000) and 00/121797 DC (CEN standard PrEN 13893 2000), Resilient floor coverings with enhanced slip resistance. An original document currently in the comment review process, publication is anticipated in April 2003.

8.9.4 Swedish Standards

The Swedish Standards Institute (SIS) is an independent, nonprofit association. The Swedish Standards Board (NSS) approves Swedish Standards, which are prefixed SS. SIS now develops few standards, instead adopting standards and working with CEN and ISO representing Sweden (see http://www.sisforlag.se/eng_default.asp (publishing)).

8.9.4.1 SS 92 35 15

Under the jurisdiction of SIS, SIS Forlag AB published *SS 92 35 15, Floorings – Determination of Slip Resistance,* in 1990. Although this standard is in Swedish, a BSI (British) translation is available. The test method is based on a SATRA-type machine (see Section 8.10.2).

8.9.5 Australia/New Zealand Standards

In Australia, most standards are published by Standards Australia (SA), which is the trading name of Standards Australia International Limited, a company limited by guarantee (see http://www.standards.com.au). It is an independent, nongovernment organization; however, through a Memorandum of Understanding SA is recognized by the Commonwealth Government as the peak nongovernment Standards body in Australia, and represent Australia in ISO.

Standards Australia was founded in 1922, originally called the Australian Commonwealth Engineering Standards Association, becoming the Standards Association of Australia in 1929, and incorporated under a Royal Charter in 1951. In 1988, the named was changed to Standards Australia, and in 1999 it became Standards Australia International Limited. Currently, over 6000 Standards are maintained by approximately 9000 voluntary experts serving on around 1700 technical committees, supported by a full-time staff of 280.

As they are issued by a nongovernmental organization, AU Standards have no independent authority. Many of them are called up in Federal or State legislation, however, and then become mandatory.

Standards Australia derives 97% of its revenues from normal commercial activities and dividends from QAS Pty Ltd, a certification subsidiary. The remaining 3% represents fees for service from the Commonwealth Government for activities in the national interest (primarily international standardizing activities).

As part of the Closer Economic Relations agreement, Standards Australia maintains strong links with Standards New Zealand, with whom there is a formal agreement for preparing and publishing joint Standards where appropriate. Standards Australia has a policy of adopting International Standards wherever possible, in line with Australia's obligations under the World Trade Organization's Code of Practice, which requires the elimination of technical standards as barriers to international trade. Approximately one-third of current Australian standards are fully or substantially aligned with international standards.

8.9.5.1 The Standards Process

A request for initiating activity on a standard is initiated by industry or government, and the public support is determined before work begins. Actual committee members are selected by the representative association and not by Standards Australia. Draft standards are available to the public along with a two-month public comment period. Publication requires the support of 67% of the committee or 80% of those voting (whichever is less), with no major dissenting interest.

8.9.5.2 Australian Standards

Committee BD/94 Slip Resistance of Flooring Surfaces is a joint committee of Standards Australia and Standards New Zealand.

Australian standards specify the use of three instruments: pendulum, Tortus, and ramp test. CSIRO (see Section 8.10.3), the leading nongovernmental testing organization in Australia is the sole owner of the complex and costly ramp facilities required for testing.

8.9.5.2.1 AS/NZS 4586:1999

AS/NZS 4586:1999 is the *Slip Resistance Classification of New Pedestrian Surface Materials standard.* Prepared by a joint standards committee of Australia and New Zealand, Committee BD/94, Slip Resistance of Floor Surfaces, this standard is a partial replacement (Part 1: Requirements) to AS/NZS 3661.1:1993 *Slip Resistance of Pedestrian Surfaces.* It calls for the pendulum (e.g., BPST) using TRRL or 4S rubber for wet testing, specifying a minimum of 0.4. Floors measuring less than 0.04 receive a ZG rating, meaning the floors are not slip resistant and the risk of slipping when wet is very high.

The dry floor friction test method called for is the floor friction tester (e.g., Tortus) using 4S rubber for dry testing. Floor that have been tested by the dry method and that have not been tested wet with the pendulum receive a Z rating, meaning the "contribution of the floor surface to the risk of slipping when wet is very high."

The standard also includes the wet/barefoot ramp test (e.g., DIN barefoot ramp test) and oil-wet ramp test (e.g., DIN oil-wet ramp test), as well as a classification system for the results, based on the test method employed. The Building Code of Australia (BCA) has called up this standard, making it a legally binding document.

8.9.5.2.2 AS/NZS 3661.1:1993

AS/NZS 3661.1:1993 is the standard for *Slip Resistance of Pedestrian Surfaces.* Although AS/NZS 4586 replaces a portion of this standard, the remainder having to do with existing floor surfaces, remains in force until DR 99447 CP (the companion standard for existing pedestrian surfaces) is approved.

8.9.5.2.3 AS/NZS 4663:2002

AS/NZS 4663:2002 is the *Slip Resistance Measurement of Existing Pedestrian Surfaces* standard. Released in early 2002, this document replaces the remainder of AS/NZS 4586. Similar in many ways to AS/NZS 4586, it specifies a pendulum instrument for wet testing (using 4S or TRRL rubber, prepared with 400-grit sandpaper), and the Tortus device for dry testing (using 4S rubber prepared with 400-grit sandpaper). The ramp tests are excluded because the focus of the standard is evaluation of existing, already installed walkway surfaces (e.g., *in situ*), including surface applications and treatments. The standard indicates that it may be unsuitable for measuring some walkway surfaces such as highly profile surfaces. It indicates that slip resistance testing of carpets used for synthetic sporting surfaces is covered in AS/NZS 2983.4.

8.9.5.2.4 AS/NZS 3661.2:1994

AS/NZS 3661.2:1994 is the *Slip Resistance of Pedestrian Surfaces – Guide to the Reduction of Slip Hazards* standard. Originally published in New Zealand as NZS 5841.1—1988, the purpose of this document is to provide guidance on selection, installation, and maintenance of walkway surfaces in residential, commercial, and public areas.

8.9.5.2.5 HB 197:1999

HB 197:1999 is an Introductory Guide to the Slip Resistance of Pedestrian Surface Materials. This handbook provides guidelines for the selection of walkways surfaces as classified by AS/NZS 4586. In part, this publication provides recommendations on appropriate classifications for various types of locations, and includes a commentary on the test methods specified in 4586. It is published in concert with CSIRO (see Section 8.10.3).

8.9.5.2.6 AS/NZS 2983.4:1988

AS/NZS 2983.4:1988 is the standard for *Methods of Test for Synthetic Sporting Surfaces – Test for Slip Resistance (Method 4: Test for Slip Resistance).* This standard specifies a method for testing the slip resistance of a synthetic sporting surface. It is included herein, and it is referenced by AS/NZS 4663:2002 and AS/NZS 4586.

8.9.5.2.7 AS/NZS 1141.42:1999

AS/NZS 1141.42:1999 is the standard for *Methods for Sampling and Testing Aggregates – Pendulum Friction Test.* This standard discusses the use of a pendulum tester to establish skid resistance for roadways. It is included herein as it is referenced by AS/NZS 4663:2002 and AS/NZS 4586.

8.9.6 Canadian Standards

Developing, maintaining and implementing Canadian standards is done by the National Standards System (NSS). The Standards Council of Canada (SCC), a federal Crown corporation established in 1970 by an act of Parliament, is responsible for coordination and oversight of the NSS, which includes about 350 member organizations and 15,000 participants. The NSS has four accredited national Standards Development Organizations (SDO). To achieve and maintain accreditation, SDOs must develop consensus standards that adhere to the principles used in Canada governing the consensus process and comply with criteria established for approval of National Standards of Canada.

Committees with collective interests, which provide a balance of representation of producers, consumers, and others with relevant interests, develop the National Standards of Canada. The balance requirement, though vague, states that "… no single category of interest representation can dominate the voting procedures …".

The four Canadian SDOs are:

- Canadian Standards Association (CSA), also known as CSA International (http://www.csa.ca)
- Canadian General Standards Board (CGSB) (http://w3.pwgsc.gc.ca/cgsb)

- Bureau de normalization du Quebec (BNQ) (http://www.criq.qc.ca/bnq)
- Underwriters Laboratories of Canada (ULC) (http://www.ulc.ca)

8.9.6.1 CAN2-75.1-M77

CAN2-75.1-M77 is a slip resistance standard for wood products commonly used for decks (wet and dry).

8.9.6.2 25.1 NO.30.1-95-CAN/CCSB

25.1 NO.30.1-95-CAN/CCSB is the standard for *Methods of Sampling and Testing Waxes and Polishes Slip Resistance.* This is a "dual-designated standard," or an adoption of ASTM D2047-93 under the Waxes and Polishes Standards Committee, and is the responsibility of Public Works and Government Services Canada (PWGSC).

8.9.7 Italian Standards

8.9.7.1 DM 14 Guigno 1989 n. 236

As with most European countries, Italy measures pedestrian slip resistance as dynamic coefficient of friction (DCOF). This is a law specifying that measurement of the DCOF should be performed using the tortus (see Section 8.6). It specifies 0.40 as a threshold of safety.

8.9.8 International Organization For Standardization (ISO)

The International Organization for Standardization (ISO) (http://www.iso.ch/iso/en/ISOOnline.frontpage) is a worldwide federation of national standards bodies from 140 countries, one from each country. ISO is a nongovernmental organization established in 1947. ISO's work results in international agreements that are published as International Standards. To date, ISO's work has resulted in some 12,000 International Standards.

A corps of 30,000 volunteers in 2850 technical committees, subcommittees, and working groups carry out the technical work of ISO. The major responsibility for administrating a standards committee is accepted by one of the national standards bodies that make up the ISO membership. The member body holding the secretariat of a standards committee normally appoints one or two persons to do the technical and administrative work.

A member body of ISO is the national body in a country that is "most representative of standardization in its country." Only one such body for each country is accepted for membership of ISO. Member bodies are entitled to participate and exercise full voting rights on any technical committee and policy committee of ISO. Each member body interested in a subject has the right to be represented on a committee. Governmental and nongovernmental international organizations, in liaison with ISO, also take part in the work.

ANSI is a founding member of and the U.S. representative of ISO. ANSI participates in 78% of all ISO technical committees, and is responsible for appointing U.S. Technical Advisory Groups (TAGs), whose primary purpose is to develop and communicate U.S. positions on activities and ballots.

8.9.8.1 ISO Standards Process

To obtain final approval of a draft International Standard requires approval by two-thirds of the ISO members that have participated actively in the standards development process, and approval by 75% of all members that vote. Whether a member country votes for or against passage of an ISO standard, there is no requirement to actually implement any ISO standard as a national standard.

Through the Vienna Agreement, ISO and CEN have agreed to share work in progress, and have provisions for one or the other development standards for both. About 25% of ISO standards originate with CEN, and about 40% of CEN standards originate with ISO. This historic agreement was made between ISO and CEN for several reasons, the most salient of which were:

1. The defection of western European national standards bodies and associated manpower from ISO in favor of CEN, thus resulting in a shortage of technical expertise for ISO; and
2. ISO obtaining "buy-in" and participation from the major world market segment of the EU and avoiding duplication of work effort.

It is important to understand that 80% of all ISO technical committees have 50% or more voting members from CEN and CEN affiliated countries. ASTM has noted that ISO committees with CEN secretariats reduce ISO efforts until CEN work projects are completed. This suggests an intention to produce a completed CEN standard that can be moved through ISO with the procedural advantages offered by the Vienna Agreement.

8.9.8.2 ISO Concerns

The biases built into the ISO structure raise several concerns:

- Through the Vienna agreement, CEN standards are permitted to go to final ballot (e.g., fast-track procedure), thus limiting the extent of changes that can be made in the document. This gives CEN members a strong advantage over other ISO members, including the U.S. and Australia.
- Each country member of CEN is also a member of ISO, and that CEN requires its members to vote with CEN. Due to this large and solid voting block of 18, there is an inherent advantage for CEN standards to pass. There is also an inherent disadvantage to ISO members such as the U.S. and Australia, should CEN direct members to vote against their positions. Given these circumstances, it would appear more appropriate for CEN to have a single voting interest in ISO.

- The process tends to dilute the work of more advanced country members because standards must be suitable for less advanced country members. This can result in standards of less significant technical merit.
- Because the purpose of ISO is to promote trade, it is difficult to balance the political implications of a given standard in each country with the technical soundness and appropriateness of the standard.

8.9.8.3 ISO Slip Resistance Related Standards

8.9.8.3.1 EN 1341 (Publication 2000)

EN 1341 is the standard for *Slabs of Natural Stone for External Paving-Requirements and Test Methods*. This test method specifies the use of a pendulum tester for measuring external walkways. The U.K. EN 1341 (BS), German version EN 1341 (DIN), and other member countries ballot the identical standard.

8.9.8.3.2 EN 1342 (Publication 2000)

EN 1342 is the standard for *Setts of Natural Stone for External Paving-Requirements and Test Methods*. This test method specifies the use of a pendulum tester for measuring external walkways. The U.K. EN 1342 (BS), German version EN 1342 (DIN), and other member countries ballot the identical standard.

8.9.8.3.3 ISO 7176-13:1989

ISO 7176-13:1989 is the standard for *Wheelchairs — Part 13: Determination of Coefficient of Friction of Test Surfaces*.

8.10 OVERSEAS ORGANIZATIONS INVOLVED IN SLIP RESISTANCE

8.10.1 The U.K. Slip Resistance Research Group

Rapra Technology, Ltd. established the U.K. Slip Resistance Research Group (UKSRRG) in 1986. Ostensibly, the initial goal of this group was to develop a single standard rubber to be used for slipmeters used in the U.K. From that first objective, the group has continued to evolve, with their mission including other aspects of slip resistance measurement.

There are currently 24 members, primarily related to flooring and associated industries. Because it was conceived and controlled by a trade group organization, the UKSRRG tends to promote materials manufactured by the trade group. Membership in the UKSRRG is by invitation only, and their deliberations are not made public.

Rapra Technology was formerly the Rubber and Plastics Research Association (RAPRA), a trade group of the rubber manufacturing industry, established in 1919. Some of their research in the field of pedestrian slip resistance is conducted for and funded by the Health and Safety Executive (HSE), the British equivalent of OSHA; however, this work is often not available to the public.

Any organization can purchase membership to Rapra, which has an extensive library of technical papers relating to slip resistance issues available for a nominal fee to members only. For more about Rapra Technology, see http://www.rapra.net.

8.10.2 SATRA Footwear Technology Center, Ltd.

SATRA Technology Centre (http://www.satra.co.uk/), an independent research and technology organization for footwear and other consumer product industries, is similar in some ways to Underwriters Laboratories. Formerly the Shoe and Allied Trades Research Association, SATRA currently employs 190 scientists, technologists and support staff and serves more than 1500 member companies in 70 countries. Its main objective is to increase the profitability of its members by offering them exclusive access to research, products and services.

SATRA has played a major role in developing national and international standards for safety footwear, assessing products against the standards and providing technical support and assistance to manufacturers (see Figure 8.5). With the introduction of European CE marking, SATRA has been involved in developing European standards for safety and protective footwear through CEN Technical Committee TC161. SATRA is the leading Notified Body for CE marking of safety footwear.

Since 1974, SATRA has conducted much research in the field of slip resistance. The SATRA Whole-Shoe Tester™ is used by much of the footwear industry (see Figure 8.5). A sophisticated laboratory instrument, SATRA offers testing services and also markets the device for sale. SATRA developed test method SATRA TM 144:1999 (formerly PM144) for measuring dynamic coefficient of friction, which specifies a threshold of 0.4 under wet or dry conditions for safety footwear.

In 2002, the SATRA Floor Coverings Test Division announced the development of a portable floor test instrument. Although few details have been released to date, it is based on principles similar to the laboratory machine using smooth or patterned test feet of 4S rubber. No information has been obtained regarding validation of the instrument, its reproducibility, or repeatability. As of this writing, the apparatus is not commercially available.

8.10.3 Commonwealth Scientific and Industrial Research Organization (CSIRO)

Australia's Commonwealth Scientific and Industrial Research Organisation (CSIRO) (http://www.dbce.csiro.au/) is an independent statutory authority created and operated

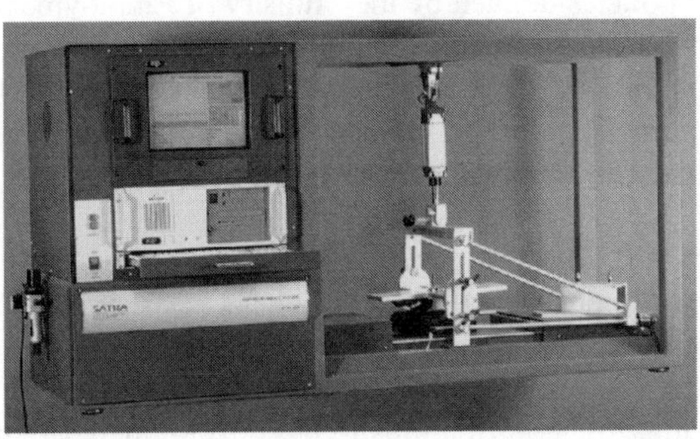

FIGURE 8.5 The SATRA whole-shoe slip resistance tester (STM603). Photograph courtesy of SATRA.

under the provisions of the Science and Industry Research Act 1949. CSIRO is an agency in the Industry, Science and Resources government portfolio and provides independent expert advice to the government, and thus is influential in forming policy relating to science and technology.

CSIRO Australia has a staff of more than 6000, conducts some 10% of Australia's total R&D effort, including about 12% of the research and development (R&D) contracted out by industry. Globally, CSIRO is active in more than 70 countries with over 700 current or recently completed projects. For the 2000–2003 triennium, the Federal Government has invested $1.5 billion in CSIRO's R&D portfolio.

CSIRO's income for 1998–1999 was $728.3 million — 65% from Parliament, 35% from outside sources, such as competitive granting schemes and research funded by industry and others, and earned revenue. CSIRO enters into commercial arrangements private and public organizations for such transactions as contract research, commercial licensing, and consulting and technical services. The Built Environment Sector, under which slip resistance issues fall, is one of 22 CSIRO Sectors.

CSIRO employs a variety of slip resistance testing equipment including the German ramp tester, British pendulum (Stanley and Wessex), (Tortus and Gabbrielli) floor friction testers, ASTM C1028 horizontal dynamometer pull meter, Whiteley HPS, and the SATRA STM 603 slip resistance tester.

The Australian Tile Council, as the "official" laboratory for determining product quality and resolving industry disputes, recognizes CSIRO.

8.10.4 INRS National Research and Safety Institute

The INRS is a nonprofit organization (http://www.inrs.fr/index_fla.html), created in 1947 under the auspices of the CNAMTS. It was originally named Institut National de Sécurité (INS, National Safety Institute) and took on its current name, Institut National de Recherche et de Sécurité (INRS, National Research and Safety Institute), in 1968. With a staff of about 600, the INRS operates on behalf of the employees and companies coming under the general Social Security scheme.

Its budget of about 400 million French francs comes almost entirely from the National occupational accident and disease prevention fund. Its activities are programmed in accordance with directives from the National salaried workers' health insurance fund and policies defined by the Ministry of Employment and Solidarity. A joint board of directors, representing employers and employee trade unions, manages it.

Regarding slips and falls, INRS has a standing committee known as A.4 Hazards Associated with Falling (Persons or Objects). Among other research, this committee has done work in the following areas, mostly in French:

- Analysis of 600 *in situ* slip resistance measurements
- The slippage of footwear and surfaces — what measurement techniques to use
- Analysis of measurements of slip resistance of soiled surfaces on site
- Comparison of seven methods for the evaluation of the slip resistance of floor coverings — contributions to the development of standards
- The prevention of slipping accidents — a review and discussion of work related to the methodology of measuring slip resistance

8.10.5 WFK Research Institute for Cleaning Technology

WFK is a German nonprofit, member-based society promoting pre-competitive research in the field of cleaning technologies for textile and non-textile materials, including hard surface cleaning (http://www.wfk.de/). The Cleaning and Maintenance Techniques Research Association (FRT) supports many projects. Much of their material is in the process of being translated from German to English, including information on slip resistance and COF.

8.10.6 Berufsgenossenschaftliches Institut fur Arbeitssicherheit (BIA)

BIA is the primary research and testing organization in Germany for statutory accident insurance and prevention (http://www.hvbg.de/d/bia/starte.htm). Their work also involves certification of products and quality management systems. Their database of approximately 1100 technical publications include several relating to slip resistance, and all are available at no charge by mail or by downloading from the BIA Web site. Although the database is searchable in English, French, and Spanish, many publications are currently in available only in German. Slip resistance research papers include work related to walkway surfaces and footwear, some using proprietary apparatus that is not well known outside of Germany developed such as the GMG 100 and the Schuster Machine (both dragsled class instruments), as well as ramp tests.

8.10.7 Finnish Institute of Occupational Health (FIOH)

FIOH is a research and advisory institute for occupational health and safety (http://www.occuphealth.fi/e/). With a total of 850 employees, 10 health and safety disciplines are covered, providing services to all of Finland. Among the research projects undertaken by FIOH are the evaluation of the slip resistance of footwear and floor surfaces, slips on ice, and methods of reducing slipping accidents. These projects are funded by various organizations, and some are done in collaboration with other organizations such as SATRA and INRS. FIOH also offers testing and certification services for slip resistance of footwear and walkway surfaces.

8.10.8 National Occupational Health and Safety Commission (NOHSC)

NOHSC is a cooperative effort of government, industry, and employee representatives (http://www.nohsc.gov.au/). A semigovernmental body of Australia, its mission is to lead and coordinate national efforts to prevent workplace injuries. Slip and fall accidents are a major concern; therefore, NOHSC has initiated a number of studies in this area. These include investigation into more realistic tests for slip resistance, flooring safety, factors of slip and fall accidents, and footwear slip resistance measurement.

8.10.9 International Association of Athletics Federations (IAAF)

The International Association of Athletics Federations was founded in 1912 by 17 national athletic federations who saw the need for a governing authority, for an athletic program, for standardized technical equipment and world records (http://www2.iaaf.org/TheSport/Technical/Tracks/Appendix4.html). The number of affiliated federations grew from 17 in 1912 to 210 in 1999. The IAAF is headquartered in Monaco and staffed by over 40 full-time, multinational professional staff. The IAAF has used corporate sponsorship as a means to better promote and develop the sport worldwide. In 2001, the IAAF Congress voted unanimously for the organization's name to be changed to the International Association of Athletics Federations.

The IAAF Performance Specifications for Synthetic Surfaced Athletics Tracks, under Section 1.6 of Specifications, specifies the use of a pendulum tester (Skid Resistance Tester). It sets a threshold for synthetic surface friction of no less than 0.5 wet, corresponding to a 47 reading on the pendulum. Appendix 4 of this Specification deals with the two acceptable methods of measuring friction.

- Method A provides instructions for measuring friction using the pendulum.
- Method B specifies the use of the Stuttgart Sliding Test apparatus (or SST), an obscure and arcane device of large size and little note (see Section 8.9.2).

EXHIBIT 8.1
NATIONAL STANDARDS BODIES

Although it is not comprehensive, the following is a listing of many national standards bodies. Not all have activity related to slip resistance or fall prevention. Note that websites and memberships are subject to change.

Algeria
Institut Algerien de normalization (IANOR)
No Web site
Membership: ISO

Argentina
Argentine Institute of Standards (IRAM)
http://www.iram.com.ar/home_es.htm (No English)
Membership: COPANT, ISO

Armenia
Department for Standardization, Metrology and Certification (SARM)
No Web site
Membership: ISO

Australia
Standards Australia (SA)
http://www.standards.com.au (English)
Membership: ISO

Austria
Osterreichisches Normungsinstitut (ON)
http://www.on-norm.at/index_e.htm (English, partial)
Membership: CEN, ISO

Bangladesh
Bangladesh Standards and Testing Institution (BSTI)
No Web site
Membership: ISO

Barbados
Barbados National Standards Institute (BNSI)
No Web site
Membership: COPANT

Belarus
State Committee for Standardization, Metrology and Certification of Belarus (BELST)
No Web site
Membership: ISO

Belgium
Institut Belge de Normalisation/Belgisch Instituut voor Normalisatie (IBN/BIN)
http://www.ibn.be/ (English, partial)
Membership: CEN, ISO

Bolivia
Bolivia Institute of Quality and Standards (IBNORCA)
http://www.boliviacomercio.org.bo/ibnorca (No English)
Membership: COPANT

Bosnia and Herzegovina
Institute for Standards, Metrology and Intellectual Property of Bosnia and Herzegovina (BASMP)
http://www.bih.net.ba/%7Ezsmp (No English)
Membership: ISO

Botswana
Botswana Bureau of Standards (BOBS)
No Web site
Membership: ISO

Brazil
Brazilian Association of Technical Standards
http://www.mre.gov.br/cdbrasil/itamaraty/web/ingles/economia/ctec/pesqind/abnt/
Membership: COPANT

Bolivia
Instituto Boliviano de Normalizacion y Calidad
http://www.boliviacomercio.org.bo/ibnorca (No English)
Membership: COPANT, ISO

Bulgaria
State Agency for Standardization and Metrology (BDS)
No Web site
Membership: ISO

Canada
Standards Council of Canada
http://www.csa-intl.org (English)
http://www.pwgsc.gc.ca/text/home-e.html (English)
Membership: COPANT, ISO

Chile
Instituto Nacional de Normalizacion (INN)
http://www.inn.cl/index.html (No English)
Membership: COPANT, ISO

China
China State Bureau of Quality and Technical Supervision (CSBTS)
http://www.csbts.cn.net/english/index.htm (English)
Membership: ISO

Colombia
Instituto Colombiano de Normas Tecnicas y Certificacion (ICONTEC)
http://www.icontec.org.co/(No English)
Membership: COPANT, ISO

Costa Rica
Costa Rica Institute of Technical Standards (INTECO)
http://www.inteco.or.cr/index1.htm (No English)
Membership: COPANT, ISO

Croatia
State Office for Standardization and Metrology (DZNM)
http://www.dznm.hr/indexen.html (English)
Membership: ISO

Cuba
National Office of Standards (NC)
No Web site
Membership: COPANT, ISO

Cyprus
Cyprus Organization for Standards and Control of Quality (CYS)
No Web site
Membership: ISO

Czech Republic
Czech Standards Institute (CSNI)
http://www.csni.cz/ (No English)
Membership: ISO

Denmark
Dansk Standard (DS)
http://www.ds.dk/(No English)
Membership: ISO

Dominican Republic
Main Directorate of Standards and Quality Control Systems (DIGENOR)
No Web site
Membership: COPANT

Ecuador
Ecuador Institute of Standardization (INEN)
Membership: COPANT, ISO

Egypt
Egyptian Organization for Standardization and Quality Control (EOS)
No Web site
Membership: ISO

El Salvador
Nacional Council of Science and Technology of El Salvador (CONACYT)
http://www.conacyt.gob.sv/(No English)
Membership: COPANT

Ethiopia
Quality and Standards Authority of Ethiopia (QSAE)
No Web site
Membership: ISO

Finland
Finnish Standards Association (SFS)
http://www.sfs.fi/english.html (English)
Membership: CEN, ISO

France
Association Francaise de Normalisation (AFNOR)
http://www.AFNOR.fr/portail.asp?Lang=English
Membership: CEN, ISO

Germany
Deutsches Institut fur Normung e.V. (DIN)
http://www.en.din.de (English, Partial)
Membership: CEN, ISO

Ghana
Ghana Standards Board (GSB)
No Web site
Membership: ISO

Greece
Hellenic Organization for Standardization (ELOT)
http://www.elot.gr/home.htm (English)
Membership: CEN, ISO

Grenada
Grenada Bureau of Standards (GDBS)
No Web site
Membership: COPANT

Guatemala
Guatemalian Commission of Standards (COGUANOR)
No Web site
Membership: COPANT

Guyana
Guyana National Bureau of Standards (GNBS)
http://www.sdnp.org.gy/gnbs/(English)
Membership: COPANT

Honduras
Honduran Council of Science and Technology (COHCIT)
Membership: COPANT

Hong Kong, China
Innovation and Technology Commission (ITCHKSAR)
http://www.info.gov.hk/itc/eng/about/mission_and_values.shtml (English)
Membership: ISO

Hungary
Magyar Szabvanyugyi Testulet (MSZT)
http://www.mszt.hu/Angol/indexeng.htm (English)
Membership: ISO

Iceland
Icelandic Council for Standardization (STRI)
Membership: CEN, ISO

India
Bureau of Indian Standards (BIS)
http://www.bis.org.in/
Membership: ISO

Iran, Islamic Republic of
Institute of Standards and Industrial Research of Iran (ISIRI)
http://www.isiri.org/
Membership: ISO

Iraq
Central Organization for Standardization and Quality Control (COSQC)
No Web site
Membership: ISO

Ireland
National Standards Authority of Ireland (NSAI)
http://www.nsai.ie/index.html (English)
Membership: CEN, ISO

Israel
Standards Institution of Israel
http://www.sii.org.il:81/neweng/eng.htm
Membership: ISO

Italy
Ente Nazionale Italiano di Unificazione (UNI)
http://www.uni.com/eng/index.shtml (English)
Membership: CEN, ISO

Jamaica
Jamaica Bureau of Standards (JBS)
No Web site
Membership: COPANT, ISO

Japan
Japanese Industrial Standards Committee (JISC)
http://www.jisc.go.jp/eng/
Membership: ISO

Kazakhstan
Committee for Standardization, Metrology and Certification (KAZMEMST)
http://www.memst.kz/(No English)
Membership: ISO

Kenya
Kenya Bureau of Standards (KEBS)
http://www.kebs.org/(English)
Membership: ISO

Korea, Democratic People's Republic
Committee for Standardization of the Democratic People's Republic of Korea (CSK)
No Web site
Membership: ISO

Korea, Republic of
Korean Agency for Technology and Standards (KATS)
http://www.ats.go.kr/English/eng_home.asp
Membership: ISO

Kuwait
Standards and Industrial Services Affairs (KOWSMD)
No Web site
Membership: ISO

Libyan Arab Jamahiriya
Libyan National Centre for Standardization and Metrology (LNCSM)
No Web site
Membership: ISO

Luxembourg
Service de l'Energie de l'Etat (SEE)
http://www.etat.lu/SEE/(No English)
Membership: CEN, ISO

Macedonia
Zavod za standardizacija i metrologija (ZSM)
No Web site
Membership: ISO

Malaysia
Standards and Industrial Research of Malaysia (SIRIM)
http://www.sirim.my/ (English)
Membership: ISO

Malta
Malta Standards Authority (MSA)
http://www.msa.org.mt/(English)
Membership: ISO

Mauritius
Mauritius Standards Bureau (MSB)
No Web site
Membership: ISO

Mexico
Nacional Office of Standards (DGN)
Membership: COPANT, ISO

Moldova, Republic of
Department of Standards, Metrology and Technical Supervision
http://www.ournet.md/~standard/en/index.htm (English)
Membership: ISO

Mongolia
Mongolian National Centre for Standardization and Metrology (MNCSN)
No Web site
Membership: ISO

Morocco
Service de normalization industrielle marocaine (SNIMA)
http://www.mcinet.gov.ma/(No English)
Membership: ISO

Netherlands
Nederlands Normalisatie-instituut (NNI)
http://www.nni.nl/nl/alg/index_afwijkend.htm (English)
Membership: CEN, ISO

New Zealand
New Zealand Standards
http://www.standards.co.nz/(English)
Membership: ISO

Nicaragua
Ministry of Development, Industry and Comerse Office of Technology, Standard and Metrology (MIFIC)
http://www.mific.gob.ni/(No English)
Membership: COPANT

Nigeria
Standards Organisation of Nigeria (SON)
http://www.sononline-ng.org/(English)
Membership: ISO

Norway
Norges Standardiseringsforbund (NSF)
Norwegian Council for Building Standardization
http://www.standard.no/index.asp?id=1533 (English) Membership: ISO

Pakistan
Pakistan Standards Institution (PSI)
No Web site
Membership: ISO

Panama
Panamian Commission of Industrial and Technical Standards (COPANIT)
http://www.mici.gob.pa/ (No English)
Membership: COPANT, ISO

Paraguay
National Institute of Technology of Standards (INTN)
No Web site
Membership: COPANT

Peru
National Institute of Defense of the Competition and the Protection of the Intellectual Property (INDECOPI)
http://www.indecopi.gob.pe/ (No English)
Membership: COPANT

Philippines
Bureau of Product Standards (BPS)
Membership: ISO

Poland
Polish Committee for Standardization (PKN)
http://www.pkn.com.pl/ (No English)
Membership: ISO

Romania
Asociatia de Standardizare din Romania (ASRO)
No Web site
Membership: ISO

Russian Federation
State Committee of the Russian Federation for Standardization and Metrology (GOST R)
http://www.gost.ru/sls/gost.nsf/PVP/CA5400452C7991BEC32566DA004601FA?OpenDocument&ALT (English)
Membership: ISO

Portugal
Instituto Portugues da Qualidade (IPQ)
http://www.ipq.pt/ (No English)
Membership: CEN, ISO

Santa Lucia
Santa Lucia Bureau of Standards (SLBS)
No Web site
Membership: COPANT

Saudi Arabia
Saudi Arabian Standards Organization
http://www.saso.org.sa/ (English)
Membership: ISO

Singapore
Singapore Productivity and Standards Board
http://www.spring.gov.sg/portal/main.html
Membership: ISO

Slovakia
Slovak Institute for Standardization (SUTN)
http://www.sutn.gov.sk/en/index2.html (English)
Membership: ISO

Slovenia
Standards and Metrology Institute (SMIS)
http://www.usm.mzt.si/English/index.htm (English)
Membership: ISO

South Africa
South African Bureau of Standards (SABS)
http://www.sabs.co.za/(English)
Membership: ISO

Spain
Asociacion Espanola de Normalizacion y Certificacion (AENOR)
http://www.aenor.es/desarrollo/inicio/home/home.asp (English)
Membership: CEN, ISO

Sri Lanka
Sri Lanka Standards Institution (SLSI)
http://www.nsf.ac.lk/slsi/
Membership: ISO

Sweden
Swedish Standards Institute (SSI)
http://www.sisforlag.se/eng_default.asp (English)
Membership: ISO

Switzerland
Swiss Association for Standardization (SNV)
http://www.snv.ch/ (No English)
Membership: CEN, ISO

Syrian Arab Republic
Syrian Arab Organization for Standardization and Metrology (SASMO)
No Web site
Membership: ISO

Tanzania, United Republic of
Tanzania Bureau of Standards (TBS)
No Web site
Membership: ISO

Thailand
Thai Industrial Standards Institute (TISI)
http://www.tisi.go.th/ (English)
Membership: ISO

Trinidad and Tobago
Trinidad and Tobago Bureau of Standards (TTBS)
No Web site
Membership: COPANT, ISO

Tunisia
Institut National de la normalization et de la propriete industrielle (INNORPI)
No Web site
Membership: ISO

Turkey
Turk Standardlari Enstitusu (TSE)
http://www.tse.org.tr/English/default.asp (English)
Membership: ISO

Ukraine
State Committee of Standardization, Metrology and Certification of Ukraine (DSTU)
http://www.dstu.gov.ua (No English)
Membership: ISO

United Arab Emirates
Directorate of Standardization and Metrology (SSUAE)
http://www.uae.gov.ae/(English)
Membership: ISO

United Kingdom
British Standards Institute (BSI)
http://www.bsi-global.com/group.xalter (English)
Membership: CEN, ISO

Uruguay
Uruguayan Institute of Technical Standards (UNIT)
Membership: COPANT, ISO

Uzbekistan
Uzbek State Centre for Standardization, Metrology and Certification (UZGOST)
No Web site
Membership: ISO

Venezuela
Standards and Quality Certification Fund (FONDONORMA)
http://www.fondonorma.org.ve/indeng.html (English, Under Construction)
Membership: COPANT, ISO

Viet Nam
Directorate for Standards and Quality (TCVN)
http://tcvn.gov.vn/
Membership: ISO

Yugoslavia
Savezni Zavod Za Standardizaciju (SZS)
No Web site
Membership: ISO

Zimbabwe
Standards Association of Zimbabwe (SAZ)
No Web site
Membership: ISO

Note: COPANT — Pan American Standards Commission; CEN — European Committee for Standardization (Comite European de Normalisation); and ISO — International Organization for Standardization

EXHIBIT 8.2
APPROACHES TO DEVELOPMENT OF STANDARDS

Consensus means that there is substantial agreement by directly and materially affected interest categories. Generally, this means concurrence of more than a simply majority (usually two-thirds), but unanimity is not required. Consensus requires that all views and objections be considered, and that an effort is made to resolve them.

There are degrees of consensus, and consensus standards can be developed in several different ways.

Full Consensus Method

Full consensus is the most open and balanced approach to standards development. For that reason, it can also be the most time-consuming and labor intensive. Full consensus requires the following elements:

"Due Process"

"Due process" requires that any person or entity with a material interest in the subject of the standard has a right to participate in the process of development and approval. Participation includes the right to express a position and its basis, have the position considered and appeal. For this reason, full consensus requires making the draft document public for a reasonable period in order to permit all interested parties the opportunity to review and comment on it.

Transparency (Openness)

Participation is open to all entities directly and materially affected by the subject of the document. There cannot be onerous financial or unreasonably restrictive technical requirements precluding the involvement of interested parties. The right to vote cannot be contingent upon membership in any organization.

Timely notice of actions regarding actions of a committee or document must be provided to all known materially affected interests. Notice must include a clear and meaningful description of the purpose of the activity and include a readily available source of additional information.

The affiliation and interest category of each member of the committee must be made available to interested parties on request.

Balance (Lack of Dominance)

The committee must have a balance of interests to preclude one interest from dominating and controlling the outcome of the process. Dominance means a position of undue influence by reason of superior leverage or representation that inhibits fair and equitable consideration of other viewpoints.

There are several methods of achieving and maintaining balance. In the case of ASTM, no more than 50% of the membership of a technical committee can be classified as producers of the subject of the standard. NFPA divides membership so that a technical committee has no more than 25% of any voting interest classification. Traditional guidelines are that no single interest category constitutes:

- More than one-third of the membership in a committee dealing with safety
- A majority of the membership in a committee dealing with product standards

Canvass Method

A step down from the full consensus methods of standards development is the canvass method. In it, certain aspects of full consensus are truncated in order to increase flexibility and reduce the time and effort needed to complete the standards process.

It appears that the canvass method was originally developed in order to have a mechanism for trade associations to be able to document existing industry practices and to have them recognized nationally. It is now used to initiate, develop, and publish standards from the ground up. The canvass method has been used to develop more than 1000 ANSI standards and about half of all ANSI-accredited organizations are approved to use this method.

The canvass method is used when a level of agreement among a drafting group has been obtained, and wider consensus is sought through a "canvass" of interested parties. Once a draft standard has been developed, the standards developer identifies, to the extent possible, entities directly and materially affected by the subject of the standard. The standards developer then conducts a letter ballot (or canvass) of those interests to determine consensus on a document.

Although the requirements of the canvass method for due process and transparency are essentially the same as in the full consensus method, two critical differences exist:

- Interested parties need not be afforded the opportunity to be involved in the process of developing the standard, only in its approval.
- Although no single interest party may dominate the canvass list, balance requirements are more readily relaxed.
- There is no requirement to adjudicate a point of view other than those held within the group. Thus, the canvassed group has no right to appeal. Only within the selected group is consensus required.

Industry Method

Unless full consensus or canvass methods are used, standards developed by an industry association or trade group usually have no requirements for due process, transparency, or balance. Because the mission of these organizations is to promote and protect their industry, these standards are often replete with inherent biases. Although an industry standard may be the product of the dictionary definition of consensus, it is the consensus of a single interest group, generally providing no opportunity for public comment. More appropriately, documents from these sources should be considered "voluntary standards" instead of "voluntary consensus standards."

9 Profiles of Selected Industries

9.1 INTRODUCTION

Hazards and exposures related to falls can vary widely depending on the type of facility. The following is a discussion of several operations that historically involve high potential for falls, by visitors, patrons, residents, and/or employees. While not a thorough discussion, these profiles attempt to cover the more common conditions contributing to falls.

9.2 ALL OCCUPANCIES

9.2.1 Exterior Controls

1. Parking lots and other exterior walking surfaces must be kept well maintained and in good repair at all times. Even small cracks or imperfections can pose a significant trip hazard to an elderly visitor to the facility.
2. Drains should be inspected on a regular basis to keep them clear and freely running. This will keep water from pooling on the surface where it can freeze.
3. Prompt snow and ice removal is essential. Gutters and downspouts should be regularly inspected to make sure they are clear of debris and do not allow water to drip or pass over any walking surfaces. Whereas water from gutters and downspouts might not pose a problem during warmer summer months, in the winter it freezes into ice and presents a serious slip and fall exposure.
4. Exterior lighting should be adequate in all areas and should be inspected and maintained on a regular basis to assure its proper functioning. Timers or photoelectric sensors should be used to ensure that exterior lights come on at dusk before total darkness sets in.
5. In the fall, leaves should be kept off of all parking lot and sidewalk surfaces. Wet leaves can present a very slippery surface if left untended.
6. Ramps should be lightly sloped and handrails should be provided.

9.2.2 Interior Controls

1. Good housekeeping practices are critical. Hallways, aisles, and stairwells, for example, should be kept clear of all unnecessary items that might pose a tripping hazard or otherwise impede the flow of foot traffic.
2. A regular floor management policy should be implemented that assigns responsibility to specific individuals to check the floors on a regular basis for dropped items, spills, damaged mats or housekeeping issues, etc.

3. A formalized spill control and cleanup program should be implemented to quickly identify and eliminate fluids from the floor surfaces.
4. Slop rugs and floor mats should be utilized during inclement weather seasons. These items should be checked regularly to make sure that edges do not curl up and present a tripping hazard, and that they do not become waterlogged. Waterlogged rugs can actually increase the hazard because people will track water off of the rug and onto the floor surface as they enter the building.

9.3 RESTAURANTS

For employees, slips and falls is the second most serious injury in the restaurant industry. They are also the most frequent, accounting for over 85% of all worker accidents, and most occur in the kitchen. Indirect costs include new employee hiring/training, overtime, and accident investigation. In terms of severity, falls represent 45% of all workers compensation claims dollars.

Restaurant, bar, and other food service operations by their very nature present a high potential for slips, trips, and falls. Increased transient foot traffic by individuals who are often unfamiliar with the exterior parking lot design or the interior layout of the building is commonplace in the industry. Guests range in age from newborn children to the very elderly, and include the physically and mentally challenged. In many cases, language and other ethnic barriers may also pose a problem. These businesses can be open "24/7," and nighttime operations are the rule rather than the exception.

Exterior parking lot areas take many shapes and configurations. Parking lots are typically subject to heavy abuse from truck traffic (either by customer trucks or by delivery and service trucks), and damaged parking lot areas are a frequent concern. Parking lot layout can play a critical role in controlling the exterior exposure. Employees dragging damaged trash bags across the parking lot area on the way to the trash dumpsters can create a significant hazard by dripping oil and food waste across pedestrian traffic paths. The presence of unique landscaping areas with walking paths, children's playground equipment, exterior stairs and balconies, and inclined ramps to building entries all heighten the exposure to slips and falls. Once inside, the customer may be faced with any of a myriad of trip, slip, and fall hazards. Multiple interior levels are often associated with steps or staircases; tables and chairs are sometimes elevated, requiring the customer to take an unaccustomed step down; highly finished dance floors may be present; and changes in floor surfaces are quite common. Dim interior lighting, the presence of alcoholic beverages, and the fact that food and drink spillage is an industry norm all can combine to heighten the interior exposure.

Employees not only face all the exposures encountered by the customers of the operation, they are also subject to the dangers in the back of the house. Wet and greasy floors are always a potential hazard. Water in the dishwashing area, oil and grease coming off of the cooking equipment, spills in the food preparation area, and ice-covered floors in the walk-in freezers are all significant slip hazards. Supplies and equipment stored in the walkways, trash waiting to be taken out, and other similar housekeeping issues are not uncommon. High employee turnover creates ongoing training and awareness issues.

9.4 HOSPITALITY (LODGING)

Hospitality operations such as hotels, motels, resorts, and casinos by their very nature present a high potential for slips, trips, and falls. Continuous foot traffic by individuals often unfamiliar with the parking lot design or the interior building layout are the norm. Guests range in age from newborn children to the very elderly, and include the physically and mentally challenged. In many cases, language and other ethnic barriers may also pose a problem. These businesses are open 24/7.

Guests and employees are exposed to a wide variety of slip, trip, and fall exposures, depending on the extent of the operation. Parking lot areas are sometimes large and confusing and incoming guests often have to maneuver through them after dark. Higher-end operations may have elaborate exterior landscaping with planted specialty walkways, bridges traversing man-made or natural streams, and unique overhead skyways. Exterior playground equipment for the smaller guests is also occasionally provided.

Inside, visitors may be exposed to an almost unlimited variety of slip, trip, and fall hazards. Large, open lobbies and common areas with sunken seating groups and changing floor surfaces increase the exposure as soon as one steps inside. Meeting rooms can be fraught with peril, from temporary electrical cord tangles and tightly packed seating conditions on poorly maintained folding chairs. In many hotel rooms, the tub is raised and the unexpected step-down causes many a headlong plunge into the sink or toilet. Many of these facilities have full-scale restaurant and lounge bar operations with multiple levels, raised furniture, highly waxed dance floors, and trendy floor coverings. Dim lighting, the presence of alcoholic beverages, as well as food and beverage spills increase the danger. Swimming pool and exercise rooms present other concerns. Water-covered tile floors in the shower rooms and along the pool edges can present a serious slip hazard if the tile has not been properly treated, and improperly designed or installed exercise equipment can create the potential for a tumble.

Employees are subject to these same exposures and more. Many of the behind-the-scenes operations present increased hazards for the average staff member. Kitchen operations at some point or another have water and grease on the floor, and stock, equipment, and trash can often block or impede the walking surface. Laundry areas also have the potential for water-slick floors and poor housekeeping. Maintenance staff members are often put at risk while performing their normal activities. Climbing ladders, performing snow and ice removal operations, and making plumbing repairs in water-soaked areas can be a part of their daily chores. High employee turnover creates ongoing training and awareness issues.

9.5 HEALTH CARE

Nursing homes and other health care occupancies present a unique set of slip, trip, and fall hazards due to the nature and needs of the residents. They also pose unusual circumstances that increase the exposure to staff and visitors. Although it would appear that the elderly or infirm residents are the greatest risk, many serious falls at health care occupancies are associated with employee activities in their daily interactions with the residents, or to the guests and visitors of the facility, many of whom themselves are often elderly individuals visiting loved ones. Most of the standard slip, trip, and fall controls apply to everyone who steps foot on the property, while other more specific controls must be employed to meet the individual needs of patients, staff, and visitors.

Many of the residents of these facilities are slowed or impaired by age or health problems. They can injure themselves by simple errors in judgment or as a result of their diminished faculties. Vision problems can make it difficult for them to distinguish changes in floor coverings or surface levels and the glare off of highly waxed floors may cause disorientation. Loss of physical body strength and the need for assistance can lead to problems if hallway handrails and bathroom grab bars are not properly maintained or appropriately mounted to accommodate the individual's height and hand preference. Placement and operation of light switches can become critical if a resident is forced to use the bathroom in the dark because he or she cannot locate or activate the switch and cannot, or will not, wait for assistance from staff members. Because some residents who cannot control their bodily functions can unintentionally create significant slip hazards, the prompt identification and cleanup of urine and other spills is critical.

From an employee standpoint, the physical job demands associated with the daily living activities of residents regularly place employees in danger of slips, trips, and falls. The transfer of residents (e.g., from bed to chair, wheelchair to toilet) requires employees to keep their footing while lifting from awkward positions, moving the residents while often off balance, and dodging the personal belongings and room furnishings that are inevitably underfoot as they go about their tasks. Many employee activities take place in environments where liquids on the floor are the norm. Assisting residents in bathing or showering activities, working in the kitchen and dining room, and handling the laundry operations all place the employee in direct contact with wet floor surfaces daily.

Finally, the needs of outside visitors and guests cannot be overlooked. Many guests are the elderly spouses or loved ones of residents, and they are often weak and infirm themselves. A higher degree of care is required for these individuals, who often fall making the short trek from their cars into the building. Once inside, they are often prone to the same physical challenges as the residents they are visiting. Other visitors to these facilities run the gamut, from groups of preschoolers who come to sing Christmas carols to paid entertainment providers such as floppy-shoed clowns and small petting zoo operators. Each brings their own unique slip, trip, and fall exposure along with them when they set foot on the property.

9.5.1 Interior Facility Controls — Residents

1. Floor coverings with bold, loud colorful patterns and colors should be avoided. These can be very disorienting to individuals with depth perception problems.
2. Highly waxed floors can produce a glare that may daze and confuse individuals with poor eyesight. Low-gloss waxes should be used and floors

should only be lightly buffed to avoid a high-sheen finish. Shades and curtains should be employed where needed to block sunlight from streaming in and reflecting off the floors.

3. Changes in floor coverings should be clearly distinguished. Moving from tile to carpet (or vice versa) can pose a significant slip or trip hazard to the elderly.
4. Adequate lighting is essential. Light switches in patient rooms and bathrooms should be marked with tapes or paints in colors contrasting to the wall background so that they do not blend into the background and are clearly visible. They should be readily accessible and function easily.
5. Bathrooms and showers should have well maintained, secure grab bars mounted strategically for use by the patient in performing their daily living activities. Handrails in hallways should be treated in a similar fashion.
6. All residents should be given a thorough orientation of the facility. They should be walked through both their room and the rest of the building and familiarized with the layout, including the location and operation of light switches, areas where floor coverings change from one surface to another, the location of handrails and grab bars, etc. If they will have access to outdoor areas such as enclosed patios, residents should have a similar orientation to these areas.
7. All residents should be evaluated as to their physical capabilities. Can they transfer themselves to and from their beds or toilet facilities? Are assistive devices necessary and mounted properly as to height and location?
8. Residents' footwear should be evaluated for fit and construction to assure that it is appropriate for the exposure. High heels, soft-bottom slippers, etc. will probably be inappropriate for the facility and can lead to serious slips and falls.

9.5.2 Interior Facility Controls — Staff

1. Kitchen exposures
2. Laundry exposures
3. Bathroom exposures
4. Maintenance staff exposures
5. Resident transfer issues

9.6 MERCANTILE

The mercantile industry, regardless of the nature of the operation, faces many of the usual issues associated with the slip, trip, and fall exposure. Although the products and the size of their operations may differ, the basic premises exposures remain the same for customer and employee.

The large exterior parking lot areas often associated with operations of this nature are one of the primary slip and fall exposures encountered. Customer foot traffic is usually heavy and the customer makeup can range from the very young to the very old, the physically fit to the unsteady and infirm. Parking lots and sidewalks in disrepair, inadequately maintained from a snow and ice removal standpoint, and insufficient lighting are leading causes of slip and fall injuries for retail operations. Other parking lot considerations that can contribute to the exposure include the presence of speed bumps, low-profile concrete car stops, and shopping carts left uncollected.

The interior design and layout of the operation can play a major role in limiting the slip and fall exposure. Floor surfaces that are not in good repair, or floor coverings that change from one form to another (carpet to tile), dramatically increase the exposure to slips and falls. Fallen merchandise or spilled liquids or food items on an otherwise clean floor can cause a serious fall. Highly stacked stock items can create a fall exposure for employees who use stools or ladders to reach them.

Poorly placed merchandise displays often present tripping hazards, as do protruding table legs or crates. The National Safety Council provides the following recommendations in this area:

- Empty racks, unused displays, and stock containers should be removed from the sales floor and stock drawers should be closed immediately after use.
- Sales items under 12 in. high should not be displayed on the floor unless in racks or large groups, and preferably not in aisles.
- Display bases and platforms for mannequins or other displays should be at least 12 in. high. For visibility, the color of the top and sides should contrast with that of the floor, and the top edge should have no overhang or lip so that the side surface will be smooth.
- Bases should not be designed with unexpected extensions that present a tripping hazard. Bases should be round or the corners should be rounded. A display should not be placed at a counter end or at a column when the diameter of the base exceeds the width of the counter or column.

9.7 TRUCKING INDUSTRY

Spectacular collisions make the evening news, but a much more common cause of injury to truck drivers involves their ongoing exposure to slips, trips, and falls. Injuries from this exposure can often be very severe, requiring in long recovery periods for the injured employee. Truck drivers face the daily challenge of simply getting in and out of their vehicles. This is often attempted while they are loaded down with paperwork, coffee cups, and other extraneous materials, making it is easy to misstep and fall. Poor training and improperly equipped or modified vehicles often contribute significantly to this exposure. The lack of adequate grab bars as well as improperly designed steps that do not provide enough traction or actually create a hazard under adverse weather conditions are common contributory factors in injuries of this nature. A similar exposure exists for those truck drivers who are responsible for securing the loads they are carrying and must climb on and over the trailers, securing chains or coverings and inspecting tie-downs. Falls from the trailer are commonplace and often more severe due to the added contributory factors of the size, shape, and positioning of the load, which can put the driver at a higher risk of injury. An additional hazard is the improper dismounting from the trailer to the ground, which greatly increases the risk of injury.

Once out of the truck, drivers are, at some point, faced with walking across customer delivery sites covered with snow and ice, slick with rain or sleet, mired in mud or muck, or simply damaged beyond repair. When the truck driver is handling a standard delivery route, they are exposed to all aspects of the industry they are serving. Falls from docks are common, as are falls inside of trailers while climbing over stock looking for delivery items. Once inside a customer building, the driver is subject to any of a number of exposures that are beyond their control, including poor housekeeping, slippery floors in walk-in coolers and freezers, and oil and grease- covered environments. Proper footwear protocols, better management controls, focused training, and the strategic use of additional equipment can greatly assist in the reduction of the slip, trip, and fall exposures associated with the trucking industry.

EXHIBIT 9.1
GUIDELINES FOR A FALL PREVENTION PROGRAM

Psychosocial Aspects of Falls (Health Care)
Denial of Aging Process

RISK	INTERVENTION	RATIONALE/KEY POINTS
1. Denial of aging process.	1.1 Counseling initiated. A. Explanation of decline in sensory, neurological and musculoskeletal function that accompanies normal aging.	1.1 Aging process includes physical limitations including decline in visual acuity, speed of walking, reaction time and balance. A. Acceptance of restrictions imposed
2. Refusal to ask for or accept assistance in getting out of bed or in going to bathroom.	2.1 Instruct residents on reasons and consequences of falls and use of assorted assistive devices.	2.1 Grab bars, shower, chairs, walkers, canes, other assistive devices. A. Use of call light/button.
3. Failure to take corrective action of environmental fall hazards.	3.1 Assist resident in assessing environment for fall hazards. A. Explain corrective actions to take. 1. Adequate illumination.	3.1 Maintains image as a capable and functional individuals. A. Guard against risk of falling. 1. Does not attempt to accomplish tasks in areas of inadequate lighting.
4. Refuses to restrict or accept assistance in activities that may no longer perform safely.	4.1 Advise resident to allow for more time to complete specific task and to identify times when risk is lowest. 4.2 Explain alternative measures resident should take to maintain present level of functioning. A. Assistive support should, while being acceptable, also bolster self-esteem.	4.1 Examples: A. Ambulating from point A to point B. B. Reaching for objects from high places. 4.2 At the same time will guard against risk of falling. A. Target modification of fall-related activities.

Fear of Falling

RISK	INTERVENTION	RATIONALE/KEY POINTS
1. Risk of falling increased because of preoccupation with falling.	1.1 Environmental correction of falling hazards. A. Adequate illumination. B. Proper handrails. C. Nonslip step surfaces. D. Proper stair climbing. E. Wearing of individual alarm devices.	1.1 Less cognitively alert to potential environmental fall hazards.
2. Avoidance of functional activities that may lead to a fall.	2.1 Minimize resident's anxiety at performing feared activity: A. Behavior resumption of feared activity. B. Psychotherapeutic intervention. C. Environmental correction. D. Elimination of hazards.	2.1 Fear of falling basis for avoidance. A. Perform activity with resident several times to gain confidence. B. Panic attacks not indicative of underlying medical problems.

EXHIBIT 9.1
GUIDELINES FOR A FALL PREVENTION PROGRAM (CONTINUED)

Cognitive Impairment (Psychological Dysfunction)

RISK	INTERVENTION	RATIONALE/KEY POINTS
1. Residents who experience cognitive impairment due to anxiety, depression, or dementia.	1.1 Treat underlying cause of anxiety or depression. A. Look for reversible causes.	1.1 Less alert to environmental fall hazards. A. Dementia, adverse drug affects, depression, visual or hearing deficits, electrolyte disturbances, hyper, hypoglycemia, dehydration, anemia, or systemic diseases.
	1.2 Remove environmental hazards. A. Provide appropriate furniture. B. Utilization of assistive devices to support ambulation.	1.2 Less able to effectively prevent a fall in progress.

Environmental Relocation

RISK	INTERVENTION	RATIONALE/KEY POINTS
1. Environmental relocation may place residents at risk.	1.1 Ensure clear understanding about need for relocation.	1.1 Cannot be maintained in own home. A. Need for protective care. B. Emotional reactions.
	1.2 Observe residents for ability to function safely in new environment. A. Knowledge of new environment.	1.2 Unfamiliar with new environment.

Attention-Seeking Behavior

RISK	INTERVENTION	RATIONALE/KEY POINTS
1. May fall in an effort to gain attention.		Residents may be lonely due to feeling abandoned in a nursing home.
	1.1 Recognize the need for attention and for the need of increased assistance.	1.1 Falling episodes may be reflective of conscious or unconscious gesture to receive help or ensure care and involvement of family.
	A. Psychotherapy.	A. Helps to deal with feelings.
	1.2 Resolve presence of relational conflicts.	1.2 Family and friends emotionally disengaging or withdrawing or decreasing contact with.
	A. Meet with family or staff members.	A. May represent focus of attention-seeking falls.
	B. Social service involvement.	
	1.3 Provide community support and activities.	1.3 Enhances feelings of accomplishment and self-sufficiency.
	A. Participation in activities.	A. Helps cope with changes in health status.

EXHIBIT 9.1
GUIDELINES FOR A FALL PREVENTION PROGRAM (CONTINUED)
Poor Compliance

RISK	INTERVENTION	RATIONALE/KEY POINTS
1. Residents are non-compliant to therapeutic recommendations by physicians.	1.1 Outline treatment plan in simple language and involve family in implementing. A. Write out all recommendations. B. Monitor progress consistently.	1.1 Residents with cognitive dysfunction may not understand or remember recommendations.
	1.2 Discuss lifestyle changes and modifications in resident's environment.	1.2 Residents may not accept underlying problems as being responsible.
	1.3 Build rapport with resident and family.	1.3 Relationship may be impaired. A. Distrust and failure to implement recommendations.
	1.4 Coordinate medical care with community services.	1.4 May improve compliance in residents lacking social supports. A. Community services may include visiting nursing homes, home health care, and social work agencies.

EXHIBIT 9.2
STADIUM-STYLE SEATING (THEATER)

INTRODUCTION

Stadium-style seating is becoming a popular form of customer seating in theaters across the country. Along with its benefit of improved visibility for customers, stadium seating may also pose some added slip, trip, and fall exposures. Listed next are some measures you can take to help minimize slip, trip, and fall loss exposures associated with stadium-style seating.

DESIGN AND USE OF HANDRAILS

Steps should be of normal design in height of each riser and the width of each step, including nosings that protrude less than 1.5 in. There should be minimum of any deviation from step to step.

Steps between the seating levels or landings should not leave any gaps or holes between the side end of the step and the nearby seats. Gaps and holes will allow patrons to misstep into these areas while they are ascending or descending the steps.

Consideration should be given to providing a short hand rail (12 to 16 in.) at each level of seats. The rail can be attached to the concrete floor at the edge of the upper seating level and then attach to the concrete of the next lower seating level at the point near the end of the seat armrest. These handrails will help give support to patrons who need this, plus the handrails will not block or protrude into the aisle area of the seats.

LIGHTING AND IDENTIFICATION

Lights or lighting strips need to be used to illuminate and identify the steps within the auditorium. Lighting strips need to be used on the top of each step and landing so that patrons can easily see the step outline as they descend. Lighting strips or louvered lighting should be used on the vertical face of each step so that each step will be illuminated while a patron is ascending the steps. There is also lighting strips inside special stair nosings that provide illumination to the patron from either direction.

In conjunction with the lighting strips the nosings and the sides of the steps should be of contrasting colors or materials to again identify the boundaries of each step.

ADDITIONAL LIGHTING AND TIMING OF LIGHTING

In general, if the steps within the auditoriums have strip lighting on both the horizontal and vertical faces of each step and landing, the steps should be readily visible and identifiable for most patrons; however, elderly patrons and others with visual problems may see the lights, but may not be able to see the steps or their feet as they contact each step.

This loss of visual acuity, especially in a theater auditorium with steps, is accelerated when the auditorium is showing the main feature and can be heightened if the actual picture has low levels of lighting. Additional lighting is usually needed, and the timing of this lighting is especially important.

Additional lighting can come from various sources, but the most beneficial would be to use wall sconces in smaller auditoriums where main aisles are either on a wall or within one row (seven seats or less) of the wall. In larger auditoriums, with multiple aisles and entrances, additional lighting should be at the ceiling level directly over the aisles. These lights will direct their illumination directly on the aisleways for their full length, without over-illuminating the rest of the auditorium.

However, it is the timing of the additional lighting that is also critical. Most house lights are left on low levels until the movie trailers begin, where they are either turned off or severely reduced in intensity. At the end of the main feature, the house lights are not usually brought up until all the feature credits have run. It is at these two times where patrons with visual impairments or reduced acuity can easily misstep and fall.

The additional lighting should be tied to the film projectors and timed so that they will stay on during all the Trailers and preliminary announcements, and reduce in intensity once the main feature is starting. This will allow latecomers to see the aisles and steps as they search for a seat to occupy. Likewise, at the end of the Main Feature, the additional lighting should be brought up as the credits start to run. Most patrons leave the auditorium right at the start of the credit run, so that bringing up the additional lighting at this time will be beneficial to all patrons as they start to exit the auditorium.

Signage

Highly visible signs should be permanently attached to the walls at the entrance to each auditorium where it will not be block by the doors or other material. Signs should state that there are steps in the auditorium, depict this with a universal type drawing, or have both to prevent misunderstandings. If possible, the signs should also tell patrons to allow time for their eyes to adjust before attempting to use the steps in the aisle ways.

Again, highly visible signs should be placed or posted at or near the ticket windows, the main entrance, or at the entrances to the hallways leading to the auditorium doors.

Verbal Warnings by Ticket Takers/Ushers

All employees, but especially ticket takers and ushers should be trained to remind and warn patrons that there are steps within the auditoriums, to "watch your step," and to allow time for patrons' eyes to adjust if they are walking in late.

Housekeeping and Maintenance

Provide extra diligence in keeping the aisle steps clear of spills or discarded items, to minimize the probability of a slip or trip. If possible, check the steps before the end of the main feature to remove or clean such problems.

Employee Orientation

Discuss the preceding information with your employee during staff meetings. New employees need to be made aware of the special exposures associated with stadium-style seating, this being accomplished during the orientation process.

It is the responsibility of each theater manager and employees to ensure that falls do not occur in the auditoriums.

10 Accident Investigation and Mitigation

10.1 INTRODUCTION

Generally, slip and fall accidents are notorious for being poorly investigated. The potential severity of slips and falls is often underestimated, and there is a tendency to attribute these types of losses to carelessness. As a result, corrective action is less likely to be identified or taken.

Although the basic principles of accident investigation can be effectively applied to this type of loss, several aspects of slip and fall accident investigation require special handling. The types of documentation and the approach to documenting physical evidence and information about the relevant management controls is unique to slip and fall accidents. Also, more than many other types of accidents, slips and falls are a frequent subject of fraud.

10.2 PITFALLS OF ACCIDENT REPORTING AND INVESTIGATION

It can often be difficult to prepare slip and fall cases for trial because adequate investigation was not performed. This can compromise your defense, and may result in significantly higher awards and legal expenses. Issues commonly found are:

- Witnesses have not been identified, or their statements were inadequately or improperly taken.
- Little information is collected at the time of the event, when conditions and recollections are still fresh.
- Pictures of the scene are not taken shortly after the incident.
- No consideration is given to the type and condition of the claimant's footwear.
- Employees have little training or instruction on responding to and handling slip and fall incidents, increasing the likelihood of litigation and aggravated injury.
- Employee statements either are not taken or taken inadequately or improperly.
- Response time does not meet internal standards, or is otherwise inadequate.

Procedures and controls should be in place to gather and document key information immediately after the event. Employees should be trained in what their roles will be in the event they must respond to an accident. Employees should be instructed to not make any statements that may imply fault.

10.3 THEORIES OF LIABILITY

Several theories of liability are put forth in a claim in order to place the moniker of liability upon management. Commonly employed theories are:

- *Failure to Comply with Code* — a physical condition, such as a stairway or ramp, that does not comply with local building code specifications
- *Failure to Correct* — the presence of an unabated hazardous condition of which management had received sufficient prior notice
- *Failure to Warn* — not advising individuals in advance of entry into a hazardous area or exposure to a hazardous condition, or giving inadequate warnings
- *Failure to Inspect or Maintain* — an inadequate safety program or non-observance of a material existing safety program specification

10.4 ACCIDENT INVESTIGATION

Most factual investigation can be scrutinized through the legal process of discovery at a later point in time. Because of this, it is essential that all factual investigation is as accurate as possible. This includes providing specific comments about the following critical areas:

- Claimant and witness information
- Information about the actual event
- Condition and design of the building components involved
- Stairs
- Handrails
- Landings
- Adequacy of lighting levels

It is strongly recommended that a standard accident investigation format, which is tailored to guide the investigator through a fall occurrence, be used. See the exhibits in this chapter for some examples.

10.4.1 CLAIMANT AND WITNESS INFORMATION

- Claimant and witness names and contact information
- The purpose for which the claimant was on the premises — Different classes of guests may be owed different standards of care. A trespasser, for example, might be afforded a lower degree of care than would an "invitee."
- The proximity and vantage point of witnesses to the event can be important in determining what they were able to observe.

10.4.2 General Occurrence Information

- Determine whether the occurrence was a slip, a trip (over something), a stumble (excessive traction), or another type of event. This will help to compare the consistency of the claimant's later version of the accident with the reported nature of the event. Thus, if the originally claimant cited a slippery surface, but later claimed the event was a trip (or physical evidence or witness statements indicate such), the validity of both assertions can be questioned.
- Determine which foot initiated the event, and if the claimant fell backward, forward, or sideways. Again, these facts can be compared with other versions of the event and the injury for consistency.
- Establish the nature of the injury, and the body parts involved.

Obtaining this type of information as soon as possible after the event can help prevent manipulation of the facts later.

10.4.3 Detailed Occurrence Information

- Establish if the claimant usually wears glasses or contact lenses, and whether they were being worn when the accident occurred. Later, you may want to determine the nature of the prescription and possible impact on the event (e.g., Is the prescription for reading or for driving?). Finally, it could be important to find out if the prescription is current. This could be a material fact, especially if the claimant had been due or overdue for a new one.
- Find out what, if anything, the claimant was carrying, and if it may have played a role in the accident. The dimensions, weight, and ease of carrying (e.g., handles) should be determined.
- Does the claimant normally take any medication or drugs? If so, find out:
  - The type of medication so the effects (e.g., drowsiness or other impairment) can be determined
  - How recently the last dosage was taken prior to the incident and the interval between the last dose and the incident
  - If medication were not taken, but should have been, because it may later be determined to have contributed to the accident
  - If illegal drugs or alcohol were used, so the police can be contacted early on to assist in the investigation
- Determine if the claimant has any physical disabilities, including those which require the use a walker, cane, or other walking aid. Establishing whether or not the aid was in use, condition, and where it landed following the incident could be meaningful to the results of the investigation.
- Of prime importance, and often undetected, is the footwear the claimant was wearing. Photographs of the shoes, including the soles and heels, can prove valuable. Important details include:
  - Type of shoe and sole

- Tread design, amount of wear, and overall condition
- Presence of contaminants

10.4.4 Location Information

Identify the following:

- Specific area where the accident occurred
- Type of floor treatment in use, schedule of application, and if it is used in accordance with manufacturer's specifications
- Construction, textures, patterns, or profiles of the flooring material
- Floor maintenance schedule, type of cleaners, date/time last performed
- Presence or absence of:
  - Foreign substances or contaminants, including snow, ice, or water accumulation, and oils, dusts, sands, and others
  - Surface irregularities and slope
  - Subtle changes in levels and other unexpected obstructions
  - Any apparent deviations from the applicable building code

If the report is about a slippery surface, it is advisable to conduct a slip resistance test of the area in the direction the claimant was traveling. This should be done prior to cleanup or other changes in the floor, and should be made part of the accident investigation report. It is important to conduct testing as soon as possible. If too much time elapses between the event date and the test date, the claimant may contend that floor surface and maintenance conditions had materially changed. The sooner in the factual investigation process that testing can be arranged, the more useful the results will be.

Photograph and diagram the site. The photograph should include a visual indicator pointing to the specific location of the incident, using a pen or other pointing device.

10.4.5 Stairs Or Ramps

Document the following:

- Direction of travel (i.e., ascending or descending)
- Specific step or steps involved
- Tread surface construction and condition
- Type and condition of nonslip tread strips
- Step geometry (stair width, riser height, tread depth, nosings)
- Stairway slope/angle
- Presence or absence of deviations in riser height of more than 3/16 in.
- Presence or absence of deviations from applicable consensus standards and building code

10.4.6 Handrails

Identify the following:

- Handrails on one or both sides of the stairway, and whether they are accessible from the most remote part of the stairs
- Handrails extending beyond the top and bottom steps
- Shape and diameter of handrail; distance from wall
- Condition of handrail and how well it is secured
- Whether the claimant was using the handrail
- Apparent deviations from applicable consensus standards and the building code

10.4.7 Landings

Identify the following:

- Landing geometry — width and length
- Rise and run (angle) of ramp lengths to and from the landing
- Whether the door swings out over the landing
- Apparent deviations from applicable consensus standards and the building code

10.4.8 Lighting

Evaluate the following:

- Impact of extreme lighting transitions (dark to light, light to dark)
- Position of lighting source(s) relative to the claimant's direction of travel
- Overall illumination levels as compared with accepted standards (Illuminating Engineering Society of North America [IESNA], National Fire Protection Association [NFPA])
- Sources of illumination that appeared to be unavailable due to maintenance, and their impact
- Automatic or manual controlled lighting activation
- Obstructions to light sources; type and condition of lighting units

10.4.9 Management/Operational Control Information

The extent and frequency of relevant management programs should be evaluated. Not only should documentation regarding the program as intended be obtained, but documentation regarding the degree of implementation as well. Depending on the circumstances of the event, controls to be evaluated may include a wide range of inspection/housekeeping and maintenance programs, training programs, lighting, construction, and special event planning (also see Chapter 2).

10.5 INCIDENT REPORTING

Why is incident reporting important? An incident can turn into a claim if not handled properly. Using incident reports can provide a larger statistical basis for determining causes of loss, thereby making your conclusions much more accurate. For instance, if 200 slip/fall claims have occurred, adding incident reports may bring your total occurrence rate to 600 — any of which could develop into a claim. A larger population of numbers leads to more reliable statistics.

Each incident report should be treated as if it were an accident report. Incidents are accidents that may have happened. As such, they should be treated, investigated, and acted upon as if they actually had occurred.

10.6 OCCURRENCE ANALYSIS

Occurrence analysis is the process of gathering all incident and accident reports to determine if any common elements exist between them. A systematic tracking system should be developed to aid in this process.

Occurrence analysis should be incorporated into your overall safety program. This type of analysis allows for a more efficient and complete method of observing and handling overall loss trends. In conjunction with implementing corrective action for each individual claim, the occurrence analysis may call for forms of corrective action broader in scope, once trends are developed at this level. For example, it may be determined that the cleaning regimen should be improved. In many instances, this should be done not only for the area in question, but as part of a global change in maintenance across all locations and areas of the operation.

Periodic occurrence analysis will also allow for the tracking of incidents in terms of frequency and severity. In addition, a facility map should be used to plot all slip/fall reports. This may provide clear indications of areas that need attention. These measures are helpful in determining whether or not the corrective action implemented is effective or not.

10.7 CLAIM MITIGATION

In terms of mitigation, management can do several things to help mitigate the loss. Demonstrating respect and empathy for the injured party and showing a sincere concern for their well-being can often reduce the potential for a lawsuit. Although care must be taken regarding the degree of assistance offered to the injured party (to avoid other liability exposures), such measures are generally of more benefit than harm. It is not uncommon to offer "comps," or complimentary services/products (e.g., gift certificates, coupons, discounts), in order to show good faith and sensitivity. Also helpful is to follow up with the injured party by telephone to inquire as to their health.

Sixty percent of individuals surveyed who lodged malpractice lawsuits against physicians indicated that they would not have brought legal action if the doctor had been more congenial and cooperative. So, if you too do not mitigate, the chances are that you may have to litigate.

10.8 FRAUD CONTROL INDICATORS

In order to combat fraud, you must first be able to identify indicators of potential fraud. Four general categories of fraud indicators are used. Keep in mind that the presence of any single indicator alone does not necessarily mean that fraud was involved. Instead, a composite of multiple factors should simply suggest further investigation of the circumstances surrounding the event and the background of the claimant.

10.8.1 Fraud — Manner of Claimant

- Overly pushy and demanding for a quick settlement
- Uncharacteristically familiar with insurance terms and procedures
- Handles all contact in person or by phone, apparently avoiding the use of means of communication that leave a traceable trail (e.g., mail, e-mail, fax)

10.8.2 General Indicators

- Claimant is a transient or an "out-of-towner" on vacation.
- An overly enthusiastic witness is at the scene of the accident.
- The owner's, manager's, or employee's account of what happened suggests a "set-up."
- The address provided by claimant or witness is a post office box or a hotel.
- There is no supporting evidence of the presence of the reported foreign substance in claims related to food spills.
- Statements between claimant and witness(es) are inconsistent.

10.8.3 Medical or Dental Fraud Indicators

- Injuries are of the subjectively diagnosed variety (e.g., headaches, nausea, inability to sleep, soft tissue injury).
- Injuries are inconsistent with the hazard or circumstances of the incident.
- Ailments appear to be chronic, persisting for several weeks or more.
- Medical or dental bills are photocopies. Third- or fourth-generation photocopies are especially suspicious.

10.8.4 Lost Earnings Fraud Indicators

- Claimant is self-employed.
- Claimant is employed by a small or unheard of business or the business address is a post office box.
- Claimant started employment shortly before the accident.

10.9 FRAUD CONTROL

Various television exposes have highlighted the fact that slip and fall fraud is rated as the third easiest and quickest way to earn $50,000 or more. Retail shopping malls, supermarkets, and other high-traffic volume occupancies are more prone to fraud, although it could be committed anywhere. In addition to a thorough accident investigation process, more business owners and property managers are installing closed-circuit television (CCTV) systems covering strategic areas of the facility. This also helps serve security needs of the business. A perpetrator will be less prone to staging an event in view of a camera. If a claim is made, the recorded event can be used to help determine whether it is fraudulent, discourage any fraudulent claims, or be used to prosecute the perpetrator.

Good incident reporting, accident investigation, housekeeping, and maintenance *all* help to control opportunities for fraud. With good management controls in place, you can help deter and defend fraudulent claims.

10.10 DOCUMENTATION

- Document *everything*. Documenting all your management controls provides the following advantages: It can provide valuable evidence that you are taking reasonable measures to exercise a prudent and reasonable degree of care. This can help stem weak lawsuits whenever your documentation is requested during the "discovery" phase. It is important that all policies and procedures that are established are observed. Fewer things hurt your case more than the claimant being able to successfully show that you had not followed your own control procedures.
- Rules, policies, and procedures need to be in writing. Dates or version numbers should indicate when updates were completed.
- The results of self-inspections need to be documented in the form of checklists or reports that include a method for providing corrective action.
- Accident reports and investigations, as discussed previously, must be clear and detailed. In some cases, months or years can go by before these records are needed — long after the event.
- Other inspection procedures and the results of such inspection, including the spill and wet program, housekeeping, sweep logs, and maintenance/repair records need to be documented to provide evidence that procedures were followed and to provide an accounting of the conditions present at that snapshot in time.
- The results of slip resistance testing should become a routine part of inspection/maintenance and accident investigation records.
- Written specifications and results of staff training and orientation contribute to demonstrating that reasonable efforts are made to ensure that the staff is prepared to perform activities required for your safety program.

10.11 STAFF ISSUES

For effective management controls and accident response and investigation, the responsibility and authority for related activities must rest in the hands of qualified and adequately trained staff. Neglecting to provide the authority can mean unnecessary delays in the correction of a hazardous condition or response to an injured person. At the same time, staff needs to be adequately supervised. Without enforcing safety policies and procedures, you run the risk that activities will not be performed properly (or at all), thus increasing the potential for lingering hazardous conditions, injury, and liability.

A periodic, independent review of policies and procedures, implementation, and the results of your loss prevention program can help identify improvements that you might not otherwise have identified.

For an extensive discussion of legal issues related to slip and fall accidents, see Turnbow, 2001.

EXHIBIT 10.1
REPORTING AND INVESTIGATION GUIDE FOR SLIPS, TRIPS, AND FALLS

ACCIDENT REPORTING & INVESTIGATION GUIDE FOR SLIPS, TRIPS & FALLS

Date of Incident:	Time of Incident:	Inside or Outside:
Location/Address:		

Claimant Information

- ❑ Name of Claimant, Address, Telephone Number
- ❑ For what purpose was the claimant on the premises?

Witness Information

- ❑ Name of Witness, Telephone Number, Address
- ❑ How close was witness to claimant?
- ❑ What position (right, left, front, behind)?
- ❑ Obtain witness statement (what did they observe?)

Occurrence Information

- ❑ Was the fall a slip or trip?
- ❑ Which foot slipped?
- ❑ Was fall backward, forward, sideways?

Describe injury & body parts (knee, ankle, shoulder, upper arm, forearm, hand, lower back, mid-back, cervical, head)

- ❑ Specify type of footwear worn by claimant
- ❑ Sole material, Heel size & material, Condition of sole

- ❑ Does claimant normally wear glasses?
- ❑ Specify type of glasses (bifocal, trifocal, normal)
- ❑ Were glasses worn at the time of the incident?

- ❑ Specify object, size, weight, & positioning of object if claimant was carrying anything (Photo).
- ❑ Where was object after the fall?

- ❑ Does claimant normally take any medication or drugs?
- ❑ Any medication taken prior to incident?
- ❑ Time interval between last dose and slip/fall incident?

Location Design & Condition Information

- ❑ Specific Area Where Incident Occurred
- ❑ Describe type of floor surface
- ❑ Describe type of floor treatment/brand.

- ❑ Foreign substances or water on the floor/stair surface?
- ❑ If so, obtain a sample.
- ❑ If known, identify/describe substance.
- ❑ Any snow/ice accumulations (if so, describe)?

- ❑ Are any cracks, bulges, potholes, protrusions, or irregularity 1/2" or more present? Describe.
- ❑ If applicable, are changes in levels clearly marked?

Stairs (if present)

- ❑ Was the claimant ascending or descending the stairs?
- ❑ Which step or steps were involved?

- ❑ Describe tread surface (slip resistant?)
- ❑ Specify width of stairs, riser heights, tread depths, & condition of stairs.

Handrails (if present)

- ❑ Are handrails on one or both sides of the stairs?
- ❑ Do they begin & end beyond the top & bottom steps?
- ❑ Specify shape & diameter
- ❑ Specify distance from nose of treads to handrail (at top & bottom steps)
- ❑ Was handrail loose at the time of or before the incident?
- ❑ Were handrails being used by the claimant before/during/after the fall?

Landing (if present)

- ❑ Specify dimensions
- ❑ Specify rise & run between adjacent landings
- ❑ Does door swing out into landing? (Specify dimensions)

Lighting Conditions

- ❑ Was claimant moving from a dimly lit area to a well lit area, or vice-versa?
- ❑ Was the light source behind or in front of the claimant?
- ❑ Specify illumination levels under same conditions
- ❑ Are lighting controls manual or automatic?

Information on Individual Completing Report

Name:	Title:	Telephone Number:
Address:		Date:

EXHIBIT 10.2
ACCIDENT INVESTIGATION GUIDE — RAMP FALL ACCIDENTS

Accident Investigation Guide

RAMP FALL ACCIDENTS

Tread Surface Composition (concrete, asphalt, carpet, other)
- ❑ Non-slip (Brushed concrete, friction strips, etc.)
- ❑ Cross cleats or grooves present?
- ❑ Results of slip resistance testing

Width of Ramp Tread Surface (edge to edge)

Slope of Ramp

_____ inches (vertical) in ______ (horizontal) inches
_____ feet (vertical) in ______ (horizontal) feet

Use of Ramp
- ❑ Pedestrian only
- ❑ Handicapped only
- ❑ Both
- ❑ Sign or warning that the ramp was only for the use of handicapped

Handrails
- ❑ Present on one or both sides
- ❑ Where was claimant with respect to handrails that were present? Handrail on their left or right?
- ❑ Was claimant using handrail?
- ❑ Diameter of handrails
- ❑ Vertical distance between handrail and ramp surface
- ❑ Any indication handrails were loose?

Size of Landings (both dimensions)
- ❑ Top
- ❑ Intermediate
- ❑ Bottom
- ❑ Does door open onto landing or ramp? (distance)

Type of Fall
- ❑ Backwards
- ❑ Forwards
- ❑ To side; left or right
- ❑ Portion of foot that slipped or tripped. (toe or heel, right foot or left foot)

Location of fall
- ❑ Where did slip or trip begin?
- ❑ Where did person end up?
- ❑ What was their body position?

Type of Injury
- ❑ Hip
- ❑ Knee
- ❑ Ankle
- ❑ Shoulder
- ❑ Arm (upper)
- ❑ Forearm
- ❑ Hand
- ❑ Lower back
- ❑ Mid-back
- ❑ Cervical (neck)
- ❑ Head

Eyewear
- ❑ Does claimant normally wear glasses?
- ❑ Type of glasses (bi-focal, tri-focal or normal)
- ❑ Were glasses being worn at time?

Footwear
- ❑ Type
- ❑ Sole material
- ❑ Heel size and material
- ❑ Available for inspecting?
- ❑ Have they been worn since the accident?
- ❑ When were they purchased?
- ❑ Did they fall off in accident?

Lighting
- ❑ Walking from a dimly lit area to a well lit area?
- ❑ Windows in the area of the fall? (location in relation to pedestrian path)
- ❑ Was the light behind or in front of the person?
- ❑ Test illumination levels
- ❑ Lighting controls manual or automatic? (dimmers?)

Witnesses
- ❑ How close were they?
- ❑ How many people?
- ❑ Were they to the right or left?

Load Carrying
- ❑ Right, left ? Arm, Shoulder?
- ❑ Where was object after fall?

Weather

EXHIBIT 10.3 ACCIDENT INVESTIGATION GUIDE — SLIPPERY SURFACES

Accident Investigation Guide

SLIPPERY SURFACES

Portion of foot that slipped
- ❑ Toe or heel
- ❑ Right foot or left foot

Fall Location
- ❑ Where did slip or trip begin?
- ❑ Where did claimant end up?
- ❑ How was the body situated oriented?

Type of Flooring
- ❑ Did the claimant just walk off a surface of a different type?
- ❑ How many steps?
- ❑ Resilient tiles or similar sheet flooring
- ❑ Ceramic
- ❑ Marble or Terrazzo
- ❑ Concrete
- ❑ Asphalt
- ❑ Carpeting
- ❑ Other

Floor Finish Product
- ❑ Samples available (testing/evidence): wax, plastic, other
- ❑ Product test results (if any)
- ❑ Manufacturers specs on use and COF
- ❑ Non-slip additive used?
- ❑ Materials and mixtures?
- ❑ Frequency of care?
- ❑ Procedures? (buffing, cleaning, finishing)
- ❑ Date last refinished prior to accident?

- ❑ Floor care:

Mat Type and Description (if any)

Type of Fall
- ❑ Backward or forwards
- ❑ To side; left or right

Type of Injury
- ❑ Hip
- ❑ Knee
- ❑ Ankle
- ❑ Shoulder
- ❑ Arm (upper)
- ❑ Forearm
- ❑ Hand
- ❑ Lower back
- ❑ Mid-back
- ❑ Cervical (neck)
- ❑ Head

Footwear

- ❑ Sole material
- ❑ Heel size and material
- ❑ Are shoes available for testing purposes?
- ❑ Have shoes been worn since the accident? How much?

Eyewear

- ❑ Does claimant normally wear glasses?
- ❑ Type of glasses (bi-focal, tri-focal, normal)
- ❑ Were glasses being worn at time?

Foreign substance (Lubricant or other material)

- ❑ Did claimant or witness see any wetness on shoe sole after fall?
- ❑ Did claimant or witness see any substance on floor before or after fall?
- ❑ Were claimants clothes moist, wet or soiled after fall?

Lighting

- ❑ Walking from a dimly lit area to a well lit area or vice versa?
- ❑ Were there any windows in the area of the fall?
- ❑ Was the light behind or in front of the claimant?
- ❑ Test illumination levels under same conditions.
- ❑ Are lighting controls manual or automatic? (dimmers, other?)

Witnesses

- ❑ How close were they?
- ❑ How many people?
- ❑ Were they to the right or left?
- ❑ Where were they in relation to the path the claimant was walking?

Load Carrying (if any)

- ❑ Right or left arm, Shoulder?
- ❑ Where was object after fall?

Weather

EXHIBIT 10.4 ACCIDENT INVESTIGATION GUIDE — STAIRWAY FALL ACCIDENTS

Accident Investigation Guide

Stairway Fall Accidents

Type of tread surface

- ❑ Wood, concrete, carpet, other
- ❑ Results of slip-resistance testing)

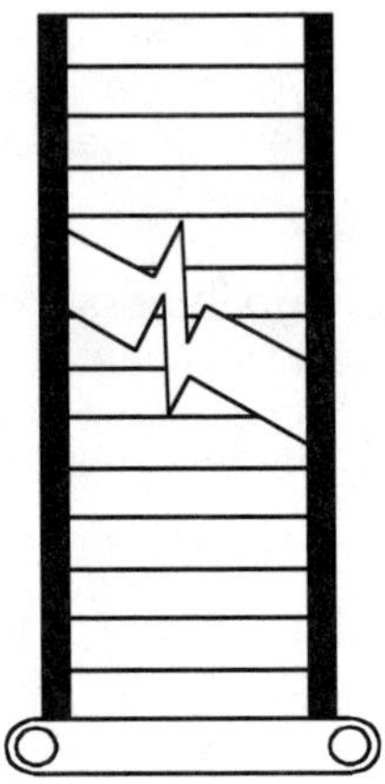

Stair Dimensions

- ❑ Width of stairs
- ❑ Riser height from top to bottom and side to side.
- ❑ Tread overhang
- ❑ Tread depth from top to bottom.
- ❑ Nosing features (Friction strips, lighting, other)

Handrails

- ❑ Do they begin and end beyond the top and bottom step.
- ❑ Is shape appropriate? Diameter?
- ❑ Distance handrail is above nose of treads at top and bottom of stairs? (should be 30-34 inches)
- ❑ Was handrail secure?
- ❑ Composition of handrails (metal, wood, other)
- ❑ Were handrails being used by the claimant?

Landings

- ❑ Dimensions
- ❑ Rise and run between adjacent landings
- ❑ Door swing out onto landing (door dimensions)

Type of fall

- ❑ A slip or trip
- ❑ What foot was it that slipped or tripped? Right, left? Was it the front foot or back foot that slipped?
- ❑ Backwards
- ❑ Forwards
- ❑ To side; left or right?

Type of Injury:

- ❑ Hip
- ❑ Knee
- ❑ Ankle
- ❑ Shoulder
- ❑ Arm (upper)
- ❑ Forearm
- ❑ Hand
- ❑ Lower back
- ❑ Mid-back
- ❑ Cervical (neck)
- ❑ Head

Type of Footwear

- ❑ Sole material
- ❑ Heel size and material
- ❑ Footwear available to examine?
- ❑ Have shoes been worn since accident?

Eyewear

- ❑ Does victim normally wear glasses?
- ❑ Type of glasses (bi-focal, tri-focal or normal)
- ❑ Were glasses being worn at time?

Lighting

- ❑ Walking from a dimly lit area to a well-lit area?
- ❑ Windows in the area of the fall? (location in relation to claimant's path of travel)
- ❑ Was the light behind or in front of the claimant?
- ❑ Test illumination levels
- ❑ Lighting controls manual or automatic (dimmers?)

Witnesses

- ❑ How close were they?
- ❑ How many people?
- ❑ Were they to the right or left?
- ❑ Load carrying
    - o Right, left? Arm, Shoulder?
    - o Where was object after fall?

Weather

Carpets or mats on the stairs, or at the top or bottom?

Bibliography

Adams, N., Slips and Falls — Some Arguments about Measuring Coefficients of Friction, *Productivity Ergonomics and Safety — The Total Package Conf.,* Gold Coast, http://www.whs.qld.gov.au/conference/ergonomic97/adams.pdf, 1997.

Adler, S.C. and Pierman, B.C., A History of Walkway Slip-Resistance Research at the National Bureau of Standards, National Bureau of Standards, Gaithersburg, MD, 1979.

Adler, S.C. and Brungraber, R., Technical Support for a Slip-Resistance Standard, ASTM STP 649, American Society for Testing Materials Standards, West Conshohocken, PA, 1978.

Alden Chemical, Why All the Confusion over Surface Types? http://www.aldonchem.com/popup-explain-surfacing-confusion.htm.

American Association of State Highway and Transportation Officials, *A Policy of Geometric Design of Highways* and *Streets*, 2001.

Andres, R.O. and Chaffin, D.B., Ergonomic analysis of slip-resistance measurement devices, *Ergonomics*, 28(7), 1065–1079 (1985).

Andrews, R.O. and Chaffin, D.B., Ergonomic analysis of slip-resistance measurement devices, *Ergonomics,* 28(7), 1065–1079 (1985).

Americans with Disabilities Act (ADA), July 26,1991, http://www.usdoj.gov/crt/ada/adahom1.htm.

A4.5 Ground and Floor Surfaces/A4.5.1 General

American National Standards Institute (ANSI), http://www.ansi.org.

ANSI Electronic Standards Store, http://webstore.ansi.org/ansidocstore/default.asp.

ANSI Procedures for the Development and Coordination of American National Standards, ANSI, March 2001.

ANSI A117.1 Standard on Accessible and Useable Buildings and Facilities.

ANSI A1264.2, Standard for the Provision of Slip Resistance on Walking/Working Surfaces, 2001.

ANSI Z41-1999, *Personal Protection — Protective Footwear.*

ANSI Z535.1, Safety Color Coding.

American Society of Mechanical Engineers (ASME), http://www.asme.org.

American Society for Testing Materials Standards (ASTM), http://www.astm.org.

ASTM, Interlaboratory Test Data for F609, Test for Static Slip Resistance of Footwear Sole, Heel, or Related Materials by Horizontal Pull Slipmeter, ASTM Research Report, West Conshohocken, PA, 1979.

ASTM C1028, Standard Test Method for Determining the Static Coefficient of Friction of Ceramic Tile and Other Like Surfaces by the Horizontal Dynamometer Pull-Meter Method

ASTM D2047, *Standard Test Method for Static Coefficient of Friction of Polish-Coated Floor Surfaces as Measured by the James Machine*

ASTM D21, Gray Pages, Book of Standards (V 15.04)

ASTM D3758 Standard Practice for Evaluation of Spray-Buff Products on Test Floors

ASTM D4103-90, *Standard Practice for Preparation of Substrate Surfaces for Coefficient of Friction Testing, 1995*

ASTM D4518-91, *Standard Test Method for Measuring Static Friction of Coating Surfaces*

ASTM D5859, Standard Test Method for Determining the Traction of Footwear on Painted Surfaces Using the Variable Incidence Tester

ASTM D6205 Standard Practice for Calibration of the James Static Coefficient of Friction Machine, 1998

ASTM E303, Method for Measuring Surface Frictional Properties using the British Pendulum Tester

ASTM F462 Standard Consumer Safety Specification for Slip-Resistant Bathing Facilities

ASTM F489, Standard Test Method for Using a James Machine

ASTM F609, Standard Test Method for Using a Horizontal Pull Slipmeter (HPS)

ASTM F695 Standard Practice for the Evaluation of Test Data Obtained by Using the Horizontal Pull Slipmeter (HPS) or the James Machine for Measurement of Static Slip Resistance of Footwear Sole, Heel, or Related Materials

ASTM F802 Standard Guide for Selection of Certain Walkway Surfaces When Considering Footwear Traction

ASTM F1240 Guide for Categorizing Results of Footwear Slip Resistance Measurements on Walkway Surfaces with an Interface of Various Foreign Substances

ASTM F1637, *Practice for Safe Walking Surfaces,* Section 7 (Speed Bumps) and Section 4.2 (Walkway Changes in Level, 1995)

ASTM F1646 Terminology Relating to Safety and Traction for Footwear

ASTM F1677-96, Standard Test Method for Using a Portable Inclineable Articulated Strut Slip Tester (PIAST)

ASTM F1678 Standard Test Method for Using a Portable Articulated Strut Slip Tester (PAST)

ASTM F1679-96 Standard Test Method for Using a Variable Incidence Tribometer (VIT)

ASTM F1694 Standard Guide for Composing Walkway Surface Evaluation and Incident Report Forms for Slips, Stumbles, Trips and Falls

ASTM F2048 Standard Practice for Reporting Slip Resistance Test Results

Architectural and Transportation Barriers Compliance Board (ATBCB), ATBCB Bulletin No.4 — Surfaces, ATBCB, Washington, DC, July 1993.

Berufsgenossenschaftliches Institut fur Arbeitssicherheit (BIA), http://www.hvbg.de/d/bia/starte.htm.

Bowman, R., The impact of new standards on the specification of tiling systems and products, Commonwealth Scientific & Industrial Research Organisation (CSIRO), Australia, 1995, http://www.infotile.com/services/techpapers/95tilex.shtml.

Bowman, R., Learning how best to live with multiple slip resistance test results, CSIRO, Australia, Revised June 1999, http://www.dbce.csiro.au/vb2/345/50/index.htm.

Bowman, R., Legal and practical aspects of problems arising from slippery floors, CSIRO, Australia.

Bowman, R., Should we recognize foreign slip resistance test results? *Tile Today*, August 2001.

Bowman, R., Slipping to your death: why it's all too-easy in Australia and what needs to be done," CSIRO, Australia, April 2000.

Bowman, R., "The Tortus floor friction tester — round robin tests," in *Ceramics, Adding the Value: AUSTCERAM 92,* M.J. Bannister, Ed., CSIRO Publications, Australia, 1992.

Bowden, F.P. and Leben, L.L., The nature of sliding and the analysis of friction, *Proc. Royal Soc. London*, 169, 371–391, 1939

Boyles, H., ASTM Committee D-21 Position Paper, ASTM Committee D-21, December 7, 1993.

Braun, R. and Roemer, D., Influence of waxes on static and dynamic friction, *Soap/Cosmetics/Chemical Specialties,* December 1974, pp. 60–72 (even).

Braun, R. and Brungraber, R.J., A Comparison of Two Slip-Resistance Testers, *ASTM STP 649*, 1978.

British Portable Skid Tester (BPST), http://www.munro-group.co.uk/skid.htm, http://www.wessexengineering.co.uk/product5.asp

British Standards Institute (BSI), http://www.bsi-global.com/group.xalter.

BS 5395, Part 1 Stairs, Ladders & Walkways. Code of Practice for the Design, Construction and Maintenance of Straight Stairs and Winders

BS 7976-1 Pendulum Testers — The Pendulum Tester Part 1: Specification

BS EN 14231 (Natural Stone) (CEN standard PrEN 14231)

BS 99/109274 DC (Ceramic Tiles and Other Rigid Tiling) (CEN standard PrEN 13552 1999)

BS 00/120903 DC (Resilient Floor Coverings) (CEN standard PrEN 13845 2000)

BS 00/121797 DC (Resilient Floor Coverings) (CEN standard PrEN 13893 2000)

Brungraber, R.J., National Bureau of Standards Technical Note 953, A New Portable Tester for the Evaluation of the Slip-Resistance of Walkway Surfaces, July 1977.

Brungraber, R.J. and Templer, J., Controlled slip resistance, *Progressive Maintenance*, March 1991, pp. 112–116.

Brungraber, R.J., English, William, Fleisher, David, Kohr, Robert, Marletta, William, Marpet, Mark, and Schieb, David, Tech news — Bucknell University F-13 workshop to evaluate various slip resistance measuring devices, *Standardization News,* May 1992, pp. 21–24.

Brungraber, R.J., personal communication to Henry Boyles, December 19, 1988.

Buczek, F.L. and Banks, S.A., High-resolution force plate analysis of utilized slip resistance in human walking, *J. Testing Evaluation,* Vol. 24, No. 6, November 1996, pp. 353–358.

Bunte, L., Traffic calming programs and emergency response: a competition of two public goods, 2000, http://www.digitalthreads.com/utarpt/utarpt5.html.

Bureau de normalization du Quebec (BNQ), http://www.criq.qc.ca/bnq.

Canadian General Standards Board (CGSB), http://w3.pwgsc.gc.ca/cgsb.

Canadian Standards Association (CSA) or CSA International, http://www.csa.ca.

CAN2-75.1-M77, Slip Resistance Standard for Wood Products Commonly Used for Decks (Wet and Dry)

25.1 NO.30.1-95-CAN/CCSB, *Methods of Sampling and Testing Waxes and Polishes Slip Resistance*

Carpet and Rug Institute (CRI), *Commercial Carpet Maintenance Manual,*

Centers for Disease Control (CDC), The costs of fall injuries among older adults, CDC, Washington, DC, January 2000.

Chandler, H., Foot Protection, "Beyond Safety Boots," OSH Canada, 2002.

Preventing Slip and Fall Injuries and Liability, *Cleaning Business Mag.,* December 1998.

Comite Europeen de Normalisation (CEN)

CEN/TC 67, http://www.cenorm.be/standardization/tech_bodies/cen_bp/workpro/tc067.htm, *PrEN 13552 (Draft) Ceramic Tiles — Determination of Coefficient of Friction*

CEN/TC 134 , http://www.cenorm.be/standardization/tech_bodies/cen_bp/workpro/tc134.htm, *PrEN 13893 — (Draft) Resilient, Laminate and Textile Floor Coverings — Parameters for the Measurement of Dynamic Coefficient of Friction on Floor Surface)*

CEN/TC 246, http://www.cenorm.be/standardization/tech_bodies/cen_bp/workpro/tc246.htm, *PrEN 14231 — (Draft) Natural Stones Test Methods — Determination of Slip Resistance by Means of the Pendulum Tester.*

PrEN 13845 — (Draft) Resilient Floor Coverings — Polyvinyl Chloride Floor Coverings with Enhanced Slip Resistance — Specification

Commonwealth Scientific and Industrial Research Organisation (CSIRO), http://www.dbce.csiro.au/.

Cramp, P., and Masters, L., "Preliminary Study of the Slipperiness of Flooring, National Bureau of Standards, 1974.

Carpet and Rug Institute, *Floor Covering Maintenance for School Facilities*, (www.carpetmaint.com).

Chemical Specialties Manufacturers Association (CSPA), Comparative Determination Slip Resistance of Floor Polishes, CSMA Bulletin No. 245–70, CSMA, 1970, Washington, D.C.

Consumer Product Safety Commission (CPSC), CPSC Product Hazard Index, Release 73–032, 1973, Washington, D.C.

Coulomb, C., Theory of simple archives, memoire de L'academie Royale Services, Vol. 10.

Davies, J.C., Kemp, G.J., Stevens, G., Frostick, S.P., and Manning, D.P., Bifocal/Varifocal Spectacles, Lighting and Missed-Step Accidents, *Safety Science,* Vol. 38, 2001, pp. 211–226.

Dravitzki, V.K. and Potter, S.M., The use of the Tortus and the pendulum with the 4S rubber for the assessment of slip resistance in the laboratory and the field, *J. Testing Evaluation,* Vol. 25, No. 1, January 1997, pp. 127–134.

Dunne, J.R., Letter to Judge Ernest F. Hollings, January 19, 1993, http://www.usdoj.gov/crt/foia/tal257.txt.

Derieux, J.B., The coefficient of friction of rubber, *J. Elisha Mitchel Scientific Society*, volume 50, p. 53–55, 1934.

Ekkebus, C., and Kiley, W., Measurement of safe walkway surfaces, *Soap, Cosmetics, Chemical Specialties,* 1973, p. 40–45.

English, W., *Pedestrian Slip Resistance: How to Measure It and How To Improve It*, 1996.

English, W., Underwood, D., and Vidal, K.E., Investigation of enhancing footwear traction for ironworkers working at heights, November 24, 1998.

English, W., "Improved Tribometry on Walking Surfaces," ASTM STP1103, 1990.

English, W., Underwood, D., and Vidal, K., Investigation of means of enhancing footwear traction for ironworkers working at heights, Occupational Safety and Safety Administration (OSHA), Washington, DC, 1998.European Committee for Standardization, http://www.cenorm.be.

Federal Register, April 1, 1990, Vol. 55, No. 69, p. 13408, 29 CFR, *Walking and Working Surfaces and Personal Protective Equipment (Fall Protection Systems); Notice of Proposed Rulemaking – Section 1910.22 General Requirements (Appendix A to Subpart D Compliance Guidelines)*

Federal Specification KK-L-115C

Federal Specification PS-624g Soap, Toilet, Liquid and Paste.

Federal Specification, Grating, Metal, Other than Bar Type (Floor, Except for Naval Vessels), RR-G-1602D, February 29, 1996.

Federal Test Method Standard No. 501a, Method 7121, *Floor Covering, Resilient, Non-Textile; Sample and Testing (Obsolete).* Federal Test Method Standard, Dynamic Coefficient of Friction, Number 501a, Method 7121, June 15, 1966.

Federal Test Method Standard No. 601, for rubber test heel and leather, Federal Specification KK-L-165 (Obsolete).

Feldman, E., The great, lowly dust mop, *Cleaning Maintenance Manage.,* January 2001.

Fendley, A.E., and Marpet, M.I., Required coefficient of friction versus walking speed: potential influences of footwear and walkway surfaces, *J. Testing Evaluation,* Vol. 24, No. 6, November 1996, pp. 359–367.

Finnish Institute of Occupational Health (FIOH), http://www.occuphealth.fi/e/.

Floor Care, Build up finish to protect VCT, December 17, 2001, http://www.cmmonline.com/ENewsArticle.asp?ArticlID = 2.

Floor Care, Long-lasting shine, long-lasting floors, March 27, 2002, http://www.cmmonline.com/ENewsArticle.asp?ArticleID = 28.

Floor Care, Top 10 signs that it's time to strip and refinish a floor," August 29, 2002, http://www.cmmonline.com/ENewsArticle.asp?ArticleID = 110.

Flynn, J.E., and Underwood, D.C., Precision and bias testing of the English XL variable incidence tribometer and the Brungraber Mark II portable inclinable articulated strut slip tester, *NOIRS 2000*, October 18, 2000.

Friedlander, M.M., P.E., CTIOA/COF report: development of safety standards for bathing facilities, Ceramic Tile Institute of American, Inc., Culver City, CA, http://www.bdf2001.com/articles/ct-bath1.htm.

Frohnsdorff, G. and Martin, M., Seeking validation and consensus on slip-resistance measurements and statistics, NIST Building & Fire Research Laboratory, Gaithersburg, MD, 1996.

German Institute for Standardization, http://www.en.din.de.

DIN 18032 P2, *Sport Halls; Halls for Gymnastics and Games; Floors for Sporting Activities; Requirements, Testing.*

DIN 51097, *Testing of Floor Coverings; Determination of the Anti-Slip Properties; Wet-Loaded Barefoot Areas; Walking Method; Ramp Test.*

DIN 51130, *Testing of Floor Coverings; Determination of the Anti-Slip Properties; Workrooms and Fields of Activities with Raised Slip Danger; Walking Method; Ramp Test.*

DIN 51131, *Testing of Floor Coverings — Determination of the Anti-Slip Properties — Measurement of Sliding Friction Coefficient.*

EN 1341 (DIN), *Slabs of Natural Stone for External Paving-Requirements and Test Methods.*

EN 1342 (DIN), *Setts of Natural Stone for External Paving-Requirements and Test Methods.*

Global Engineering Documents (GED), http://global.Ihs.com.

Gotte, T. and Heisig, A., Prevention of slipping accidents, *Die BG*, No. 9, 1999, pp. 518–523.

Goodwin, V.D., Slip and fall accidents — floor testing, March 1999, http://www.mde.cc/publications/slipfall.html.

Gray, E., Jablonsky, R., and Yoshida, H., Biomechanical measurements: pedestrian coefficient of friction, *ASTM STP 1103*, 1990.

Grieser, B., Rhoades, T., and Shah, R., Slip resistance — field measurements using two modern slipmeters, *Professional Safety,* June 2002, pp. 43–48.

Grönqvist, R., Hirvonen, M., and Rajamaki, E., Development of a portable test device for assessing on-site floor slipperiness: an interim report, *Applied Ergonomics*, 32, 2001, pp. 163–171.

Grönqvist, R., Hirvonen, M., and Tohv, A., 1999, Evaluation of three portable floor slipperiness testers, *Int. J. Industrial Ergonomics*, vol. 25, pp. 85–95.

Gronqvist, Raoul, Slips and falls, chapter 19 in *Biomechanics in Ergonomics,* Taylor & Francis, 1999, pp. 351–375.

Guevin, P.R., Status of skid and slip resistance testing relatable to painted floors, P.R. Guevin Associates.

Hanson, J., Redfern, M., and Mazumdar, M., Predicting slips and falls considering required and available friction, *Ergonomics,* 1999, vol 2, No. 12, pp. 1619–1633.

Harris, G.W. and Shaw, S.R., Slip resistance of floors: users' opinions, Tortus instrument readings and roughness measurement, *J. Occupational Accidents*, 9, 1988, pp. 298–298.

Hazardous polymerization, http://homepage.eircon.net/~safestride/index1.html.

Hedden, J., Strengthen your safety net, innovative safety programs give restauranteurs extra protection in the kitchen, 1997, http://www.restaurant.org/rusa/magArticle.cfm?ArticleID=497.

Houston, D., Paving the way for seniors, *Facilities Design Arrangement,* March 2002.

Hughes, R.C. and James, D.I., Slipping determinations — magic and myth, undated paper, RAPRA Technologies, Shawbury, Shrewsbury, Shropshire, United Kingdom.

Hunter, R.B., A method of measuring frictional coefficients of walk-way materials, *Bureau of Standards J. Res.,* pp. 329–347, 1929.

International Code Council (ICC), http://www.intlcode.org/.

ICC/ANSI A117.1, Accessible and usable buildings and facilities, 1998.

International Conference of Building Officials, http://www.icbo.org/.

Illuminating Engineering Society of North America (IESNA), *The IESNA Lighting Handbook Reference and Application,* Illuminating Engineering Society of North America, 9th ed., 2000.

IESNA, http://www.iesna.org.

Slips, Trips and Same-Level Falls, in *Industrial Safety and Occupational Health Markets,* Richard K. Miller & Associates, 5th ed., 1999, pp. 218–220.

Institut National de Recherche et de Sécurité (INRS, National Research and Safety Institute), http://www.inrs.fr/index_fla.html.

Institute for Business and Home Safety (IBHS), Summary of State-Mandated Building Codes, http://www.ibhs.org.

Institute of Transportation Engineers (ITE) Task Force TENC-5TF-01 Staff, *Guidelines for the Design and Application of Speed Humps,* ITE, Washington, DC, 1993.

International Association of Athletics Federations (IAAF), http://www2.iaaf.org/TheSport/Technical/Tracks/Appendix4.html.

International Organization for Standardization (ISO), http://www.iso.ch/iso/en/ISOOnline.frontpage.

ISO 7176-13:1989, *Wheelchairs — Part 13: Determination of Coefficient of Friction of Test Surfaces.*

Irvine, C.H., Evaluation of some factors affecting measurements of slip resistance of shoe sole materials on floor surfaces, *J. Testing Evaluation,* 1976, vol. 4, No. 2, pp. 133–138.

Irvine, C.H., Evaluation of the effect of contact-time when measuring floor slip resistance, *J. Testing Evaluation,* January 1986, vol. 14, No. 1, ASTM, pp. 19–22.

Italian Standards

DM 14 Guigno 1989 n. 236 (slip resistance as dynamic coefficient of friction)

Jablonsky, R.D., Standardization of test methods for measurement of floor slipperiness, *ASTM STP 649*, 1978.

James, D.I., A standard slider for slip measurements, *Polymer Testing,* vol. 8, 1989, pp. 9–17.

James, D.I., Assessing the slip resistance of flooring materials, *ASTM STP 1103,* 1990.

James, D.I., Slip resistance tests for flooring: two methods compared, *Polymer Testing*, 1985, vol. 5, pp. 403–425.

Jung, K. and Diecken, U., Slip resistance of floors — some critical remarks on a device used for workplace measurements, *Die BG*, No. 7, 1992, pp. 422–429.

Jung, K. and Diecken, U., Testing slip resistance of floors with the Schuster machine, *Zbl Arbeitsmedizin,* Vol. 42, No. 10, 1992.

Kime, G.A., Slip resistance and the U.K. Slip Resistance Research Group, *Safety Science,* vol. 14, 1991, pp. 223–229.

Klein, J., The extremities of safety: hand and foot protection — choosing and using safety footwear, *Compliance Mag.,* July 2002.

Liberty Mutual Insurance Company, Restaurant Floor Cleaning, 1995, http://www.libertymutual.com/research/about/1995_report/tribology-research.html.

Klik, M. and Faghri, A., A comparative evaluation of speed humps and deviations, *Transportation Quarterly,* Vol. 47, No. 3, July 1993, p. 459.

Kohr, R.L., Using ASTM slip test methods, *American Ceramic Society Bull.,* June 1995, Vol. 74, No 6., May 1992, pp. 75–78.

Krafft, L.E., Fix slopping mopping, *Cleaning Maintenance Manage.,* April 2002.

Kulakowski, B.T., Buczek, F. and Cavanaugh, P., Evaluation of performance of three slip resistance testers, *J. Testing Evaluation*, 1989, vol. 17, No. 4, pp. 234–240.

LaReau, R., Operators can build mat market on preventing slips and falls, Textile Rental Services Association (TRSA) Online, http://www.trsa.org, August 1996.

Malkin, F. and Harrison, R., Measurement of the Coefficient of Friction of Floors, *Applied Physics*, 1979, vol. 12, pp. 517–528.

Marletta, W., The effect of the use of differing sanding protocols on readings of slip resistance when using the English XL and Brungraber Mark II tribometers," Doctoral Dissertation, 1994, New York University, NY.

Marlowe, D., Letter to ASTM Technical Committee Chairmen on CEN and ISO, January 12, 2001.

Marpet, M.I., Comparison of walkway safety tribometers, *J. Testing Evaluation*, vol. 24, No. 4, pp. 245–254, 1996.

Marpet, M.I. and Fleisher, D.H., "Comparison of walkway-safety tribometers: part II, *J. Testing Evaluation,* Vol. 25, No. 1, 1997, pp.115–126.

Martin, G. and Dimopoulos, J., Reliability of dry slip resistance test results using the Tortus floor friction tester, *Productivity Ergonomics and Safety — The Total Package Conf.,* Gold Coast, http://www.whs.qld.gov.au/conference/ergonomic97/martin.pdf, 1997.

Mastrad Quality and Test Systems, http://www.mastrad.com/tortus.htm.

Maynard, W.S., Tribology: preventing slips and falls in the workplace, *Occupational Health and Safety,* 2002.

McCagg, M., Get a charge out of your equipment, *Cleaning Maintenance Manage.,* May 2002.

Medoff, H. Fleisher, D., and Di Pila, S., Comparison of slip resistance measurements between two tribometers using smooth and grooved Neolite test liner test feet, STP 1424, Metrology of Pedestrian Locomotion and Slip Resistance, ASTM International, 2003.

Miller, J.M. and Rhoades, T.P., Slip Resistance Predictions for Various Metal Step Materials, Shoe Soles and Contaminant Conditions, Society of Automotive Engineers Technical Paper Series, 1987.

Mishky, S., Lighting for improved workplace safety, *Occupational Hazards,* August 1, 2001.

Murphy, T., In search of slip-resistant flooring, *Plant Services,* March 2001.

Myung, R., Smith, J. and Leamon, T., Subjective assessment of floor slipperiness, *Int. J. Industrial Ergonomics,* 1993, vol. 11, pp. 313–319.

Nation's Restaurant News, http://www.nrn.com/operations/worksafety.html

National Building Code (NBC), http://www.bocai.org/.

National Bureau of Standards (NBS) Preliminary Study of the Slipperiness of Flooring, NBSIR 74-613, 1974.

National Occupational Health and Safety Commission (NOHSC), http://www.nohsc.gov.au/

National Safety Council (NSC), Falls on Floors, Data Sheet I-495, NSC, Itasca, IL, 1991.

NSC, *Injury Facts*, NSC, Itasca, IL, 2000.

NSC, *Injury Facts*, NSC, Itasca, IL, 1999.

NSC, *International Accident Facts*, 2nd ed., NSC, Itasca, IL, 1999.

National Fire Protection Association (NFPA), http://www.nfpa.org/.

NFPA 101, Life Safety Code, National Fire Protection Association, 2000.

NFPA 1901, Fire Equipment Apparatus, National Fire Protection Association, 1999.

NSSN: A National Resource for Global Standards, http://www.nssn.org.

Occupational Safety and Health Administration, OSHA 1910 and 1926, http://www.osha.gov.

Manlifts 1910.68(c)(3)(v)

OSHA 29 CFR Part 1910.136

1926, Subpart M on Fall Protection

1926, Subpart R — Steel Erection Regulatory (3)

Appendix B to Subpart R — Acceptable Test Methods for Testing Slip Resistance of Walking/Working Surfaces (1926.754(c)(3)). Non-Mandatory Guidelines for Complying with 1926.754(c)(3).

1926, Subpart X on Stairways and Ladders

Notice of Proposed Rulemaking — Section 1910.22 General Requirements (Appendix A to Subpart D Compliance Guidelines)

Perkins, P., Measurement of slip between the shoe and ground during walking, *ASTM STP 649*, 1978.

Powers, C.M., Kulig, K., Flynn, J., and Brault, J.R., "Repeatability and bias of two walkway safety tribometers, *J. Testing Evaluation,* Vol. 27, No. 6, 1999, pp. 368–374.

Proctor, T.D., Slipping accidents in Great Britain — an update, *Safety Science*, 16, 1993.

Proctor, T.D. and Coleman, V., Slipping, tripping and falling accidents in Great Britain — present and future. *J. Occupational Accidents,* 9, 269–285, 1988.

Rabinowicz, Ernest, Stick and Slip, *Scientific American,* May 1956, vol. 194, no. 5, pp. 109–110, 112, 115–117.

Rapra Technology, http://www.rapra.net.

Redfern, M. and Rhoades, T., Fall prevention in industry using slip resistance testing, *Occupational Ergonomics — Theory and Application,* Vol. 27, Marcel Dekker, 1996.

Rowland, F.J., James, D.J., and Hughes, R.C., Slip resistance — an overview: the work of the UK Slip Resistance Group, *Polymer Testing '95*, Volume 17, 1995.

Rosen, S., *Slip and Fall Handbook,* Parts I, II, and II, Harlow Press, 1995.

Sacher, A., Slip resistance and the James Machine 0.5 static coefficient of friction — sine qua non, *American Ceramic Society Bull.*, pp. 30–37.

Sanford, C., Help your customers prevent slip-and-falls, *Cleaning Maintenance Manage.,* July 1999.

SATRA Technology Centre, Ltd., http://www.satra.co.uk/.

Schroder, D. and Garvens, H.J., WFK slip resistance, WFK Cleaning Technology Research Institute, http://www.wfk.de/rho/slipresistance_e.html.

Severn Science, http://www.severnscience.co.uk/pages/tortus.html

Sherman, R., Role of the expert in a slip and fall lawsuit, *Professional Safety,* 1999, pp. 37–40.

Sigler, P., Calibration and Operation of the Sigler Pendulum-Impact Type Slipperiness Tester, June 27, 1949.

Sigler, P., Geib, M., and Boone, T., Measurement of the Slipperiness of Walkway Surfaces, National Bureau of Standards, NBS RP1879, Vol. 40, 1948.

The Soap and Detergent Association, Chemistry, http://www.sdahq.org.

Sotter, G., *Stop Slip and Fall Accidents,* Soner Eronenine Corporation, Mission Viejo, CA, 2000.

Southern Building Code Congress International, http://www.sbcci.org/.

Standards Australia, http://www.standards.com.au.

AS/NZS 1141.42:1999, *Methods for Sampling and Testing Aggregates — Pendulum Friction Test.*

AS/NZS 2983.4:1988 *Methods of Test for SyntheticSSporting Surfaces — Test for Slip Resistance (Method 4: Test for Slip Resistance).*

AS/NZS 3661.1:1993, *Slip Resistance of Pedestrian Surfaces.*

AS/NZS 3661.1:1993, *Slip Resistance of Pedestrian Surfaces.*

AS/NZS 3661.2:1994, *Slip Resistance of Pedestrian Surfaces — Guide to the Reduction of Slip Hazards.*

AS/NZS 3661.2:1994, *Slip Resistance of Pedestrian Surfaces — Guide to the Reduction of Slip Hazards.*

AS/NZS 3661.2: 1994, Slip Resistance Classification Of Pedestrian Surface Materials.

AS/NZS 4586:1999, *Slip Resistance Classification of New Pedestrian Surface Materials.*

AS/NZS 4663:2002, *Slip Resistance Measurement of Existing Pedestrian Surfaces.*

Draft DR 99447 CP: 1999, Slip Resistance Measurement of Existing Pedestrian Surfaces.

HB 197:1999, Introductory Guide to the Slip Resistance of Pedestrian Surface Materials.

Strandberg, L., The effect of conditions underfoot on falling and overexertion accidents, *Ergonomics*, 28(1), 1985.

Strandberg, L., Ergonomics Applied to Slipping Accidents, Ergonomics of Workstation Design, 1983.

Swedish National Road and Transport Research Institute, "Effects on Cycling of Road Maintenance and Operation," July 26, 1999, http://www.tft.lth.se/kfbkonf/5bergstromnew.PDF.

Swedish Standards Institute (SIS) *SS 92 35 15, Floorings — Determination of Slip Resistance.*

Textile Rental Services Association (TRSA), http://www.trsa.org.

Turman, D., Slip & Fall Prevention: Floor Chemical Basics, http://Foodservice.com.

Turman, D., Slip Resistant Footwear Basics, http://Foodservice.com.

Turnbow, C.E., *Slip & Fall Practice,* 2nd ed., James Publishing, Costa Mesa, CA, 2001.

Underwriters Laboratories (UL), http://www.ul.com.

U.L. 410, Slip Resistance of Floor Surface Materials, 1996.

Underwriters Laboratories of Canada (ULC), http://www.ulc.ca.

U.S. Bureau of the Census, Life Expectancy at Birth, 1996.

U.S. Bureau of the Census, Projections of the Population by Age and Sex: 1995 to 2050, 1996.

U.S. Federal Highway Administration, *Manual on Uniform Traffic Control Devices for Streets and Highways* (MUTCD), 2001, http://mutcd.fhwa.dot.gov/

U.S. General Services Administration Specification P-F-430C(1), *Finish, Floor, Water Emulsion (Obsolete)*

U.S. Military Specifications (Navy)

MIL-D-0016680C (Ships) and MIL-D-18873B, Deck Covering Magnesia Aggregate Mixture.

MIL-D-17951C (Ships), *Deck Covering, Lightweight, Nonslip, Silicon Carbide Particle Coated Fabric, Film, or Composite, and Sealing Compound.*

MIL-D-23003a(SH), *Deck Covering Compound, Nonslip, Rollable.*

MIL-D-24483A, *Nonslip Flight Deck Compound.*

MIL-D-3134J, *Deck Covering Materials, 1988.*

MIL-W-5044C, *Walkway Compound, Nonslip, and Walkway Matting, Nonslip*

U.S. Trademark Electronic Search System (TESS) - http://www.uspto.gov/web/menu/tm.html.

Vidal, K., Slips, trips and falls, in *Safety Management Handbook*, CGH, Inc., Chicago, IL, 2000.

Waltzing to the Vienna Agreement — A refresher course, ISO Bulletin, August 1998.

Webster, T., Workplace Falls, *Compensation Working Conditions,* Spring 2000.

Weller, S.C., Floor covering ills — a prescription for mat rental services, *Textile Rental,* TRSA Online, http://www.trsa.org, September 1998.

WFK Research Institute for Cleaning Technology, http://www.wfk.de/, http://www.wfk.de/rho/slipresistance_e.html.

Williams, W.D., Smith, J.A., and Draugelis, F.J., Topaka — a new device and method for measuring slip resistance of polished floors, *Soap/Cosmetics/Chemical Specialties,* July 1972, pp. 44, 47–48, 52, 60.

A Policy on Geometric Design of Highways and Streets, American Association of State Highway Transportation Officials, 4th ed., 2001.

Index

Note: Bold page numbers refer to figures.

B

C

D

E

G

H

I

J

K

L

M

N

O

P

T

Y

Z